Affordable Anti Inflammatory Diet Cookbook

Quick and Tasty Side Dishes Recipes to Enjoy your Meals

Zac Gibson

© Copyright 2021 - All rights reserved.

The content contained within this book may not be reproduced, duplicated or transmitted without direct written permission from the author or the publisher. Under no circumstances will any blame or legal responsibility be held against the publisher, or author, for any damages, reparation, or monetary loss due to the information contained within this book. Either directly or indirectly.

Legal Notice:

This book is copyright protected. This book is only for personal use. You cannot amend, distribute, sell, use, quote or paraphrase any part, or the content within this book, without the consent of the author or publisher.

Disclaimer Notice:

Please note the information contained within this document is for educational and entertainment purposes only. All effort has been executed to present accurate, up to date, and reliable, complete information. No warranties of any kind are declared or implied. Readers acknowledge that the author is not engaging in the rendering of legal, financial, medical or professional advice. The content within this book has been derived from various sources. Please consult a licensed professional before attempting any techniques outlined in this book.

By reading this document, the reader agrees that under no circumstances is the author responsible for any losses, direct or indirect, which are incurred as a result of the use of information contained within this document, including, but not limited to, — errors, omissions, or inaccuracies.

Table of Content

Bacon and Cheddar Cheese Balls 7

Cheese Roll-Ups the Keto Way 11

Cheddar Cheese Chips 12

Cardamom and Cinnamon Fat Bombs 14

No Cook Coconut and Chocolate Bars 16

Coleslaw 18

Roasted Zucchini and Pumpkin Cubes 20

Chile Casserole 22

Pickled Jalapeno 24

Naan 26

Sauteed Tomato Cabbage 28

Tender Radicchio 30

Green Salad with Walnuts 32

Jicama Slaw 34

Peanut Slaw 36

White Mushroom Saute 38

Caesar Salad 40

Cranberry Relish 42

Vegetable Tots 44

Hasselback Zucchini 46

Lime Fennel Bulb 48

Baked Garlic.. 50

Roasted Okra... 52

Broccoli Gratin 54

Cayenne Pepper Green Beans................................. 56

Lime Brussels Sprouts 58

Cabbage Bowl.. 60

Parmesan Asparagus 62

Coconut Quinoa 64

Rosemary Black Beans... 66

Oregano Green Beans.. 68

Yam Mash 70

Soft Peas 72

Mushroom Stew 74

Cheesy Broccoli 76

Glazed Broccoli 78

Cinnamon Asparagus.. 80

Spicy Cucumbers 82

Summer Salad.. 84

Tender Quinoa 85

Chickpeas Bowl 88

Beans Mash 90

Spiralized Carrot 92

Classic Barley 94

Baked Mango 96

Easy Cabbage Slaw 98

Apple Salad 100

Avocado Mash 102

Bake Endives 104

Arugula Bowl 106

Bacon and Cheddar Cheese Balls

Prep Time:
10 Minutes
Cook Time:
8 Min
Serve: 10

Ingredients:

- ½ tsp chili flakes (optional
- 5 1⁄3-oz bacon
- 5 1⁄3-oz cheddar cheese
- 5 1⁄3-oz cream cheese
- ½ tsp pepper

Directions:

1. Pan fry bacon until crisped, around 8 minutes.

2. Meanwhile, in a food processor, process remaining ingredients. Then transfer to a bowl and refrigerate. When ready to handle, form into 20 equal balls.

3. Once bacon is cooked, crumble bacon and spread on a plate.

4. Roll the balls on the crumbled bacon to coat.

Nutrition: Calories: 225.6; Fat: 21.6g; Carbs: 1.6g; Protein: 6.4g

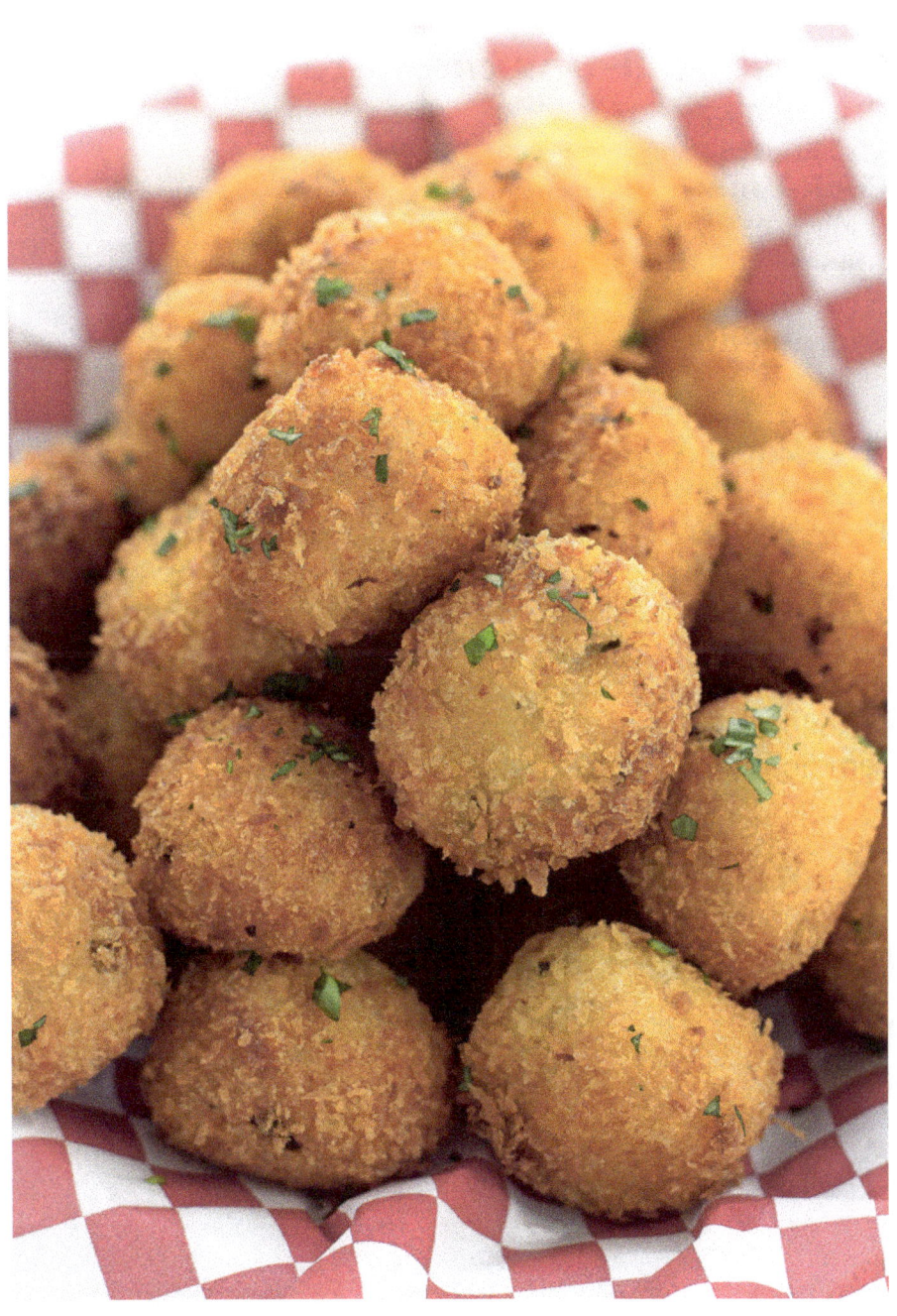

Cheese Roll-Ups the Keto Way

Prep Time:
15 Minutes
Cook Time:
0 Minutes
Serve: 4

Ingredients:

- 4 slices cheddar cheese
- 4 ham slices

Directions:

1. Place one cheese slice on a flat surface and top with one slice of ham.

2. Roll from one end to the other. Repeat process to remaining cheese and ham.

Nutrition: Calories: 60; Fat: 2.6g; Carbs: 2.5g; Protein: 6.7g

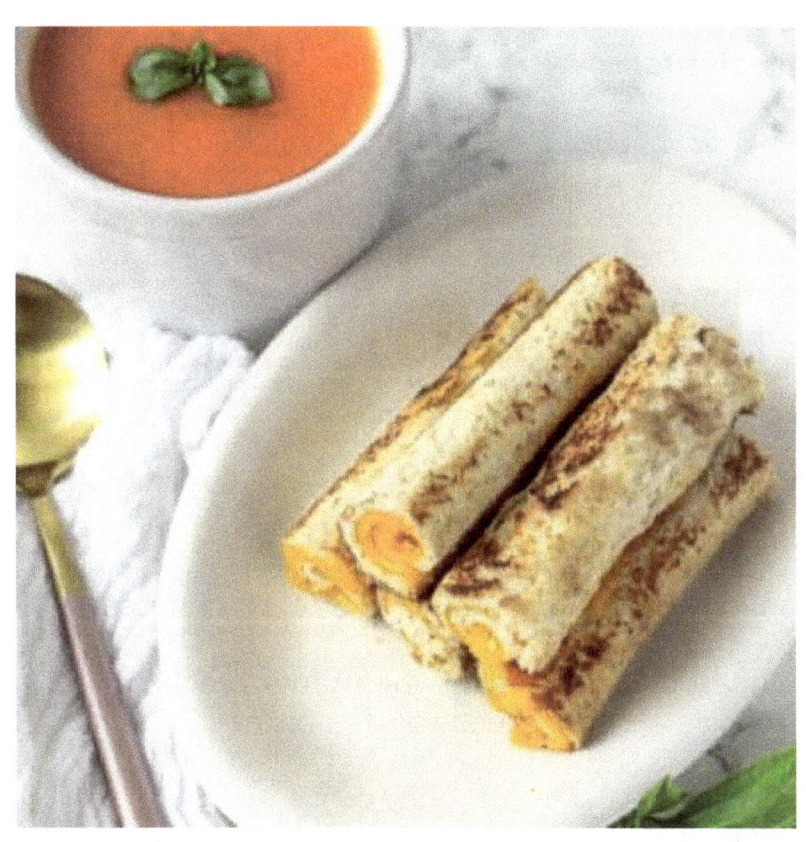

Cheddar Cheese Chips

Prep Time:
5 Minutes
Cook Time:
8 Minutes
Serve: 4

Ingredients:

- 8 oz. cheddar cheese or provolone cheese or edam cheese, in slices
- ½ tsp paprika powder None

Directions:

1. Line baking sheet with foil and preheat oven to 400oF.

2. Place cheese slices on baking sheet and sprinkle paprika powder on top.

3. Pop in the oven and bake for 8 to 10 minutes.

4. Pay particular attention when timer reaches 6 to 7 minutes as a burnt cheese tastes bitter.

Nutrition: Calories: 228; Fat: 19.0g; Carbs: 2.0g; Protein: 13.0g

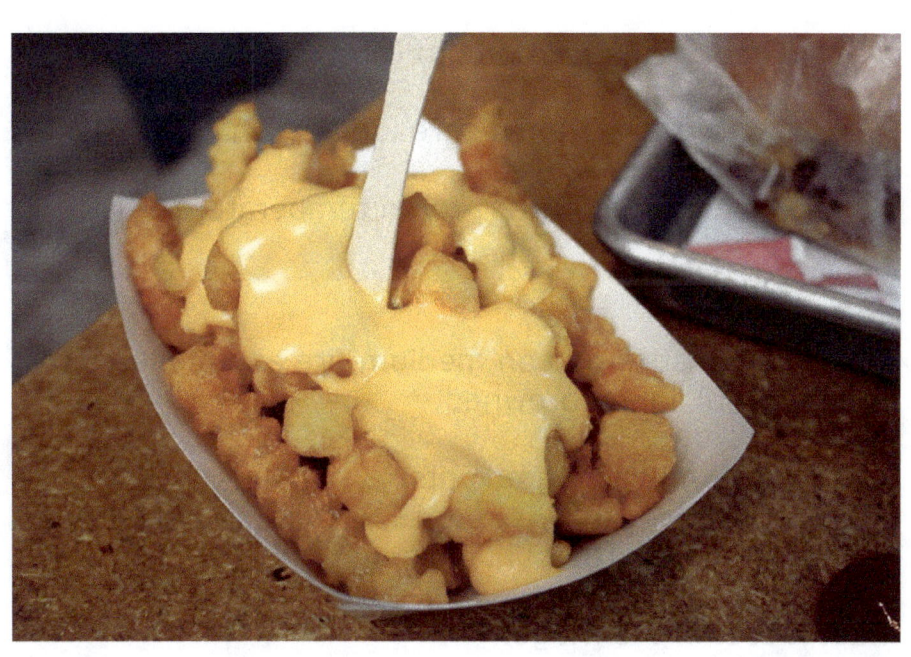

Cardamom and Cinnamon Fat Bombs

Prep Time:
5 Minutes
Cook Time:
3 Minutes
Serve: 10

Ingredients:

- ¼ tsp ground cardamom (green
- ¼ tsp ground cinnamon
- ½ cup unsweetened shredded coconut
- ½ tsp vanilla extract
- 3-oz unsalted butter, room temperature

Directions:

1. Place a nonstick pan on medium fire and toast coconut until lightly browned.

2. In a bowl, mix all ingredients.

3. Evenly roll into 10 equal balls.

4. Let it cool in the fridge.

Nutrition: Calories: 90; Fat: 10.0g; Carbs: 0.4g; Protein: 0.4g

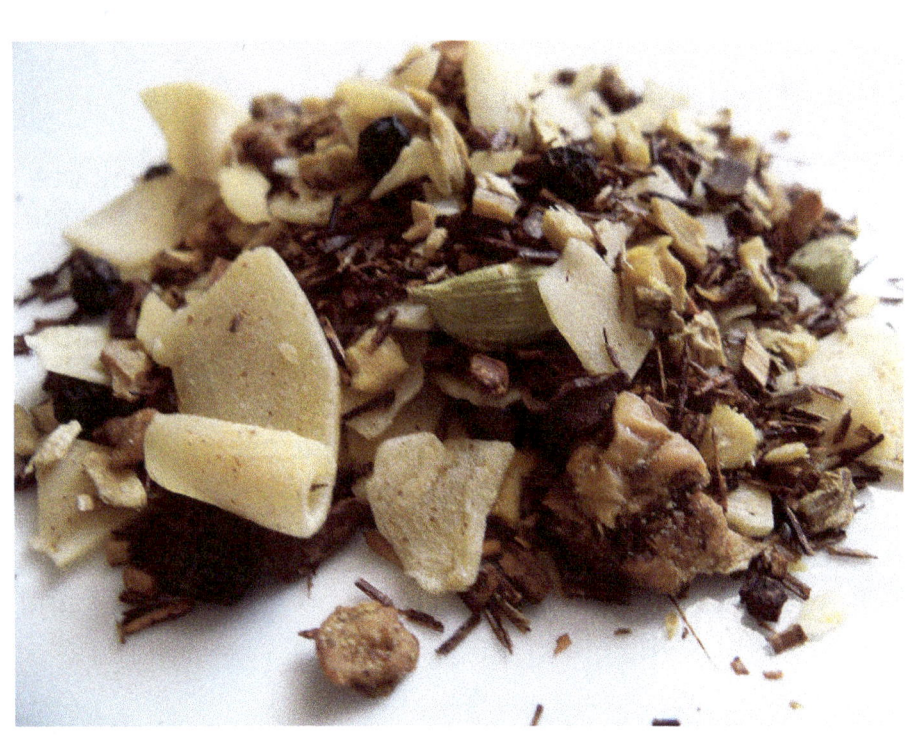

No Cook Coconut and Chocolate Bars

Prep Time:
15 Minutes
Cook Time:
0 Minutes
Serve: 6

Ingredients:

- 1 tbsp Stevia
- ¾ cup shredded coconut, unsweetened
- ½ cup ground nuts (almonds, pecans, or walnuts
- ¼ cup unsweetened cocoa powder
- 4 tbsp coconut oil Done

Directions:

1. In a medium bowl, mix shredded coconut, nuts and cocoa powder. Add Stevia and coconut oil.

2. Mix batter thoroughly.

3. In a 9x9 square inch pan or dish, press the batter and for 30-minutes place in the freezer.

Nutrition: Calories: 148; Fat: 7.8g; Carbs: 2.3g; Protein: 1.6g

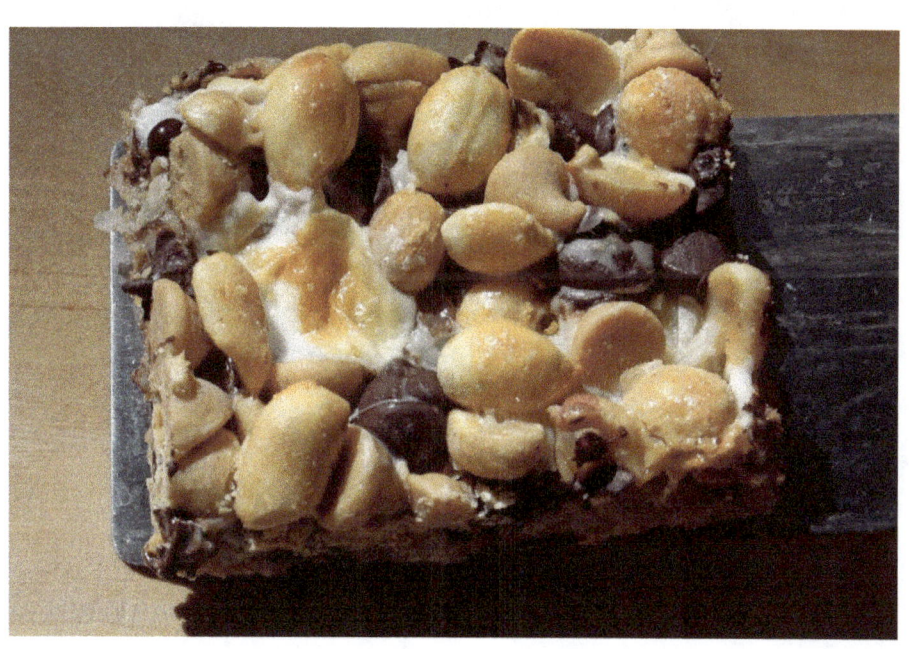

Coleslaw

Prep Time:
10 minutes
Serve: 2

Ingredients:

- 1 cup white cabbage
- 1 tablespoon mayonnaise
- ½ teaspoon ground black pepper
- ½ teaspoon salt

Directions:

1. Shred the white cabbage and place it in the big salad bowl.

2. Sprinkle it with ground black pepper and salt.

3. Add mayonnaise and mix up coleslaw very carefully.

Nutrition: calories 39, fat 2.5, fiber 1, carbs 4.1, protein 0.6

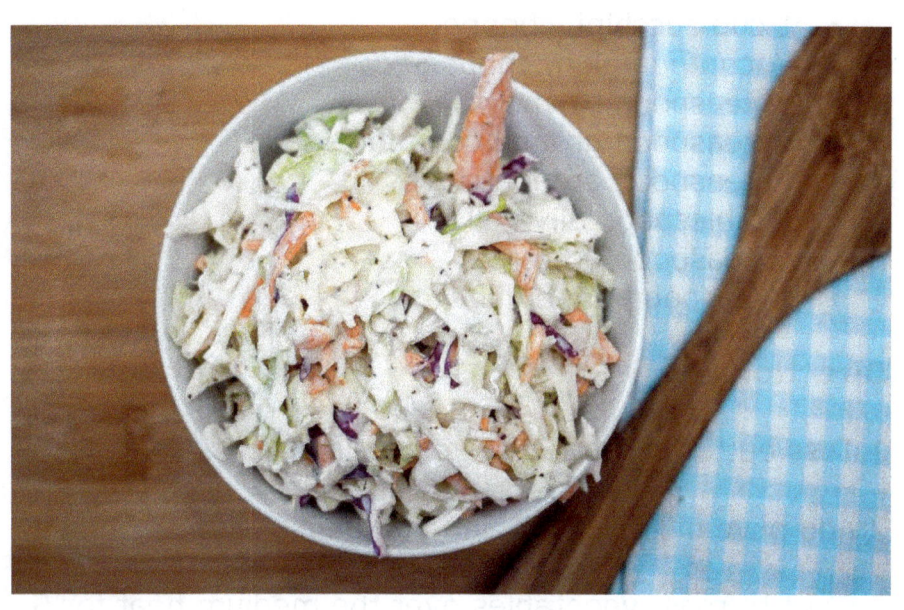

Roasted Zucchini and Pumpkin Cubes

Prep Time:
10 minutes
Cook Time:
20 minutes
Serve: 3

Ingredients:

- 1 cup zucchini, chopped
- ¼ cup pumpkin, chopped
- ¼ teaspoon thyme
- ½ teaspoon ground coriander
- ½ teaspoon ground cloves
- 1 tablespoon olive oil
- ½ teaspoon butter
- 1 teaspoon dried dill

Directions:

1. Toss butter in the skillet and melt it.

2. Add olive oil, zucchini, and pumpkin.

3. Start to roast vegetables over the medium heat for 5 minutes.

4. Hen sprinkle them with thyme, ground coriander, ground cloves, and dried dill.

5. Mix up well and close the lid.

6. Cook the vegetables on the low heat for 15 minutes.

Nutrition: calories 66, fat 5.5, fiber 1.2, carbs 3.4, protein 0.8

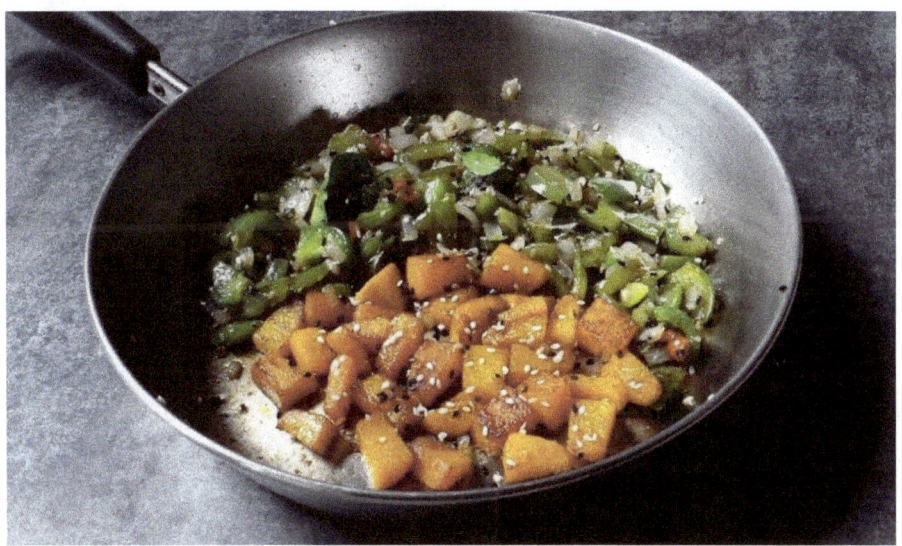

Chile Casserole

Prep Time:
15 minutes
Cook Time:
15 minutes
Serve: 4

Ingredients:

- 1 cup chili peppers, green, raw
- 1 teaspoon olive oil
- 3 oz Cheddar cheese, shredded
- 1 teaspoon butter
- 2 eggs, whisked
- ¼ cup heavy cream
- ½ teaspoon salt

Directions:

1. Preheat the grill well and place chili peppers on it.

2. Grill the chili peppers for 5 minutes. Stir them from time to time. Then chill the peppers little and peel them. Remove the seeds. Place the peppers in the casserole tray.

3. Add butter and sprinkle with salt.

4. In the separated bowl, mix up together heavy cream, whisked eggs, and cheese.

5. Pour the liquid over the chili peppers and transfer casserole in the [reheated to the 365F oven.

6. Cook casserole for 10 minutes.

Nutrition: calories 169, fat 14.2, fiber 0.3, carbs 2.4, protein 8.6

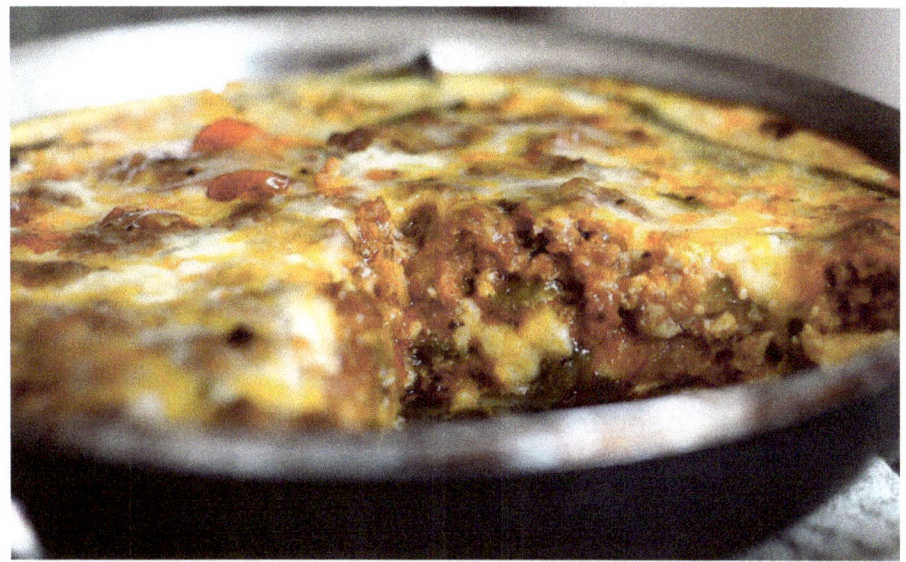

Pickled Jalapeno

Prep Time:
10 minutes
Cook Time:
10 minutes
Serve: 6

Ingredients:

- 6 jalapeno peppers
- ¼ cup apple cider vinegar
- 1/3 cup water
- ¼ teaspoon peppercorns
- 1 garlic clove, peeled
- ½ teaspoon ground coriander

Directions:

1. Pour apple cider vinegar in the saucepan.

2. Add water, peppercorns, and bring the liquid to boil. Wash the jalapeno peppers and slice them.

3. Put the sliced jalapenos in the glass jar. Add ground cinnamon and garlic clove.

4. After this, add boiled apple cider vinegar liquid and close the lid. Marinate the jalapenos as a minimum for 1 hour.

Nutrition: calories 9, fat 0.2, fiber 0.6, carbs 1.4, protein 0.2

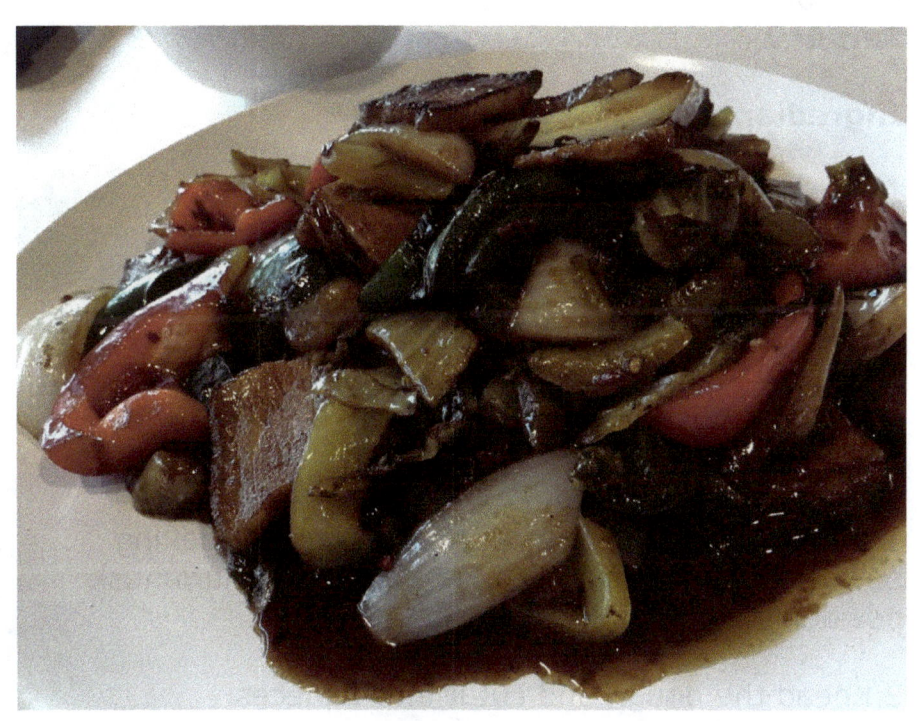

Naan

Prep Time:
10 minutes
Cook Time:
4 minutes
Serve: 2

Ingredients:

- 1 tablespoon butter
- 1 tablespoon almond flour
- ¾ teaspoon baking powder
- ¼ teaspoon lemon juice
- 1 teaspoon coconut oil, softened
- 1 teaspoon psyllium husk powder

Directions:

1. In the mixing bowl, mix up almond flour, baking powder, lemon juice, coconut oil, and psyllium husk powder.

2. Knead the dough and cut it into 2 pieces.

3. Roll up the dough pieces to get naan bread shape.

4. Toss butter in the skillet and bring it to boil.

5. Place naan bread in the preheated butter and roast for 1 minute from each side.

6. The time of cooking depends on the naan size.

Nutrition: calories 157, fat 15.1, fiber 2.7, carbs 5.2, protein 3.1

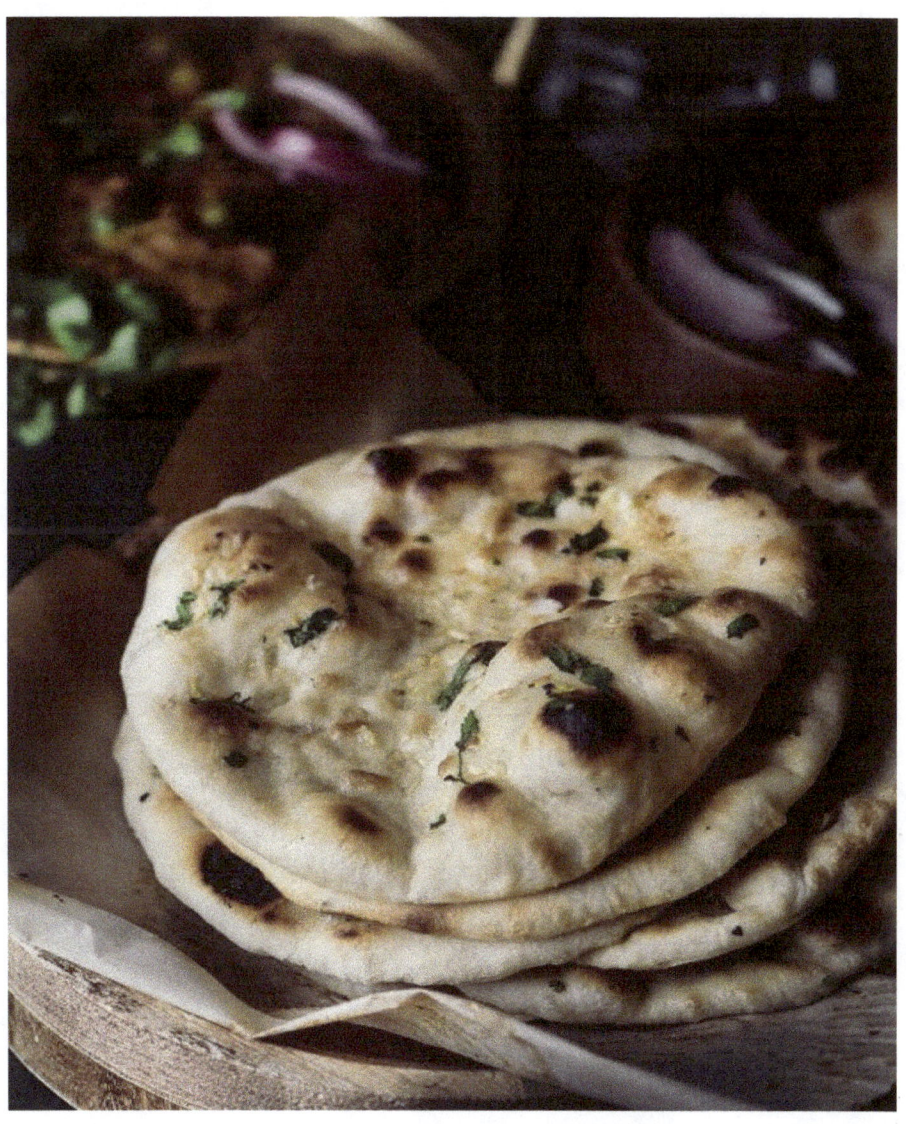

Sauteed Tomato Cabbage

Prep Time:
10 minutes
Cook Time:
35 minutes
Serve: 4

Ingredients:

- 1 tablespoon tomato paste
- 1 bell pepper, chopped
- ½ oz celery, grated
- 2 cups white cabbage, shredded
- 1 tablespoon butter
- 1 tablespoon dried oregano
- 1/3 cup water
- ¼ cup coconut cream
- 1 teaspoon salt

Directions:

1. Mix up together tomato paste, coconut cream, and water. Pour the liquid in the saucepan.

2. Add bell pepper, grated celery, white cabbage, butter, and dried oregano. Sprinkle the mixture with salt and mix up gently.

3. Close the lid and saute cabbage for 35 minutes over the medium-low heat.

Nutrition: calories 86, fat 6.7, fiber 2.3, carbs 6.7, protein 1.4

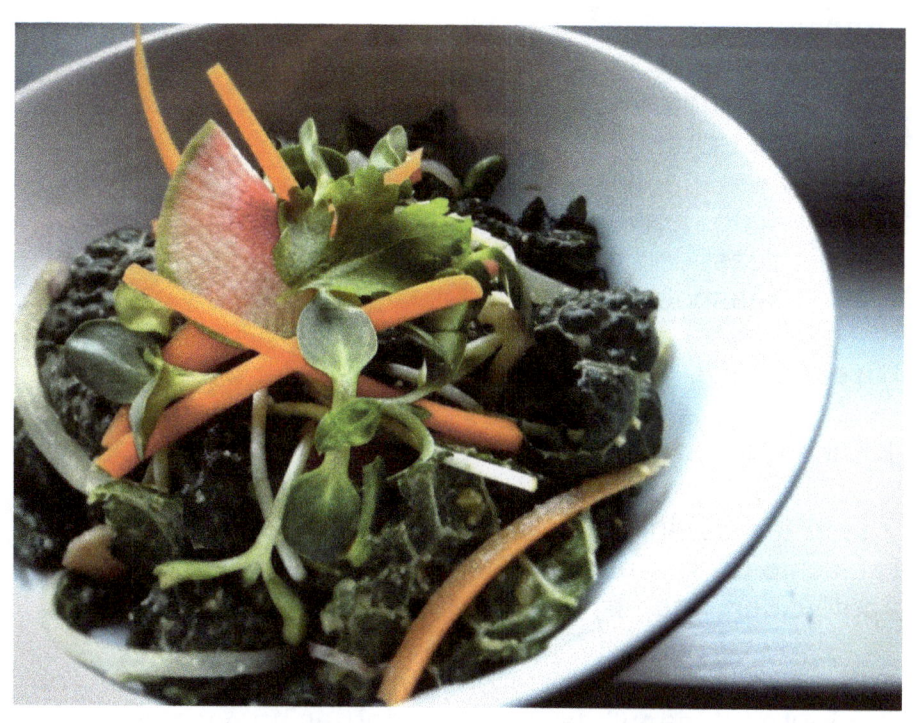

Tender Radicchio

Prep Time:
10 minutes
Cook Time:
8 minutes
Serve: 4

Ingredients:

- 8 oz radicchio
- 1 teaspoon canola oil
- ½ teaspoon apple cider vinegar
- ¼ cup heavy cream
- 1 teaspoon minced garlic
- 1 teaspoon dried dill

Directions:

1. Slice the radicchio into 4 slices.

2. Line the baking dish with parchment and put sliced radicchio on it. Sprinkle the vegetables with canola oil, apple cider vinegar, and dried dill.

3. Bake radicchio in the preheated to the 360F oven for 8 minutes. Meanwhile, whisk together heavy cream with minced garlic.

4. Transfer the cooked radicchio on the plates and sprinkle with minced heavy cream mixture.

Nutrition: calories 43, fat 4, fiber 0.2, carbs 1.5, protein 0.5

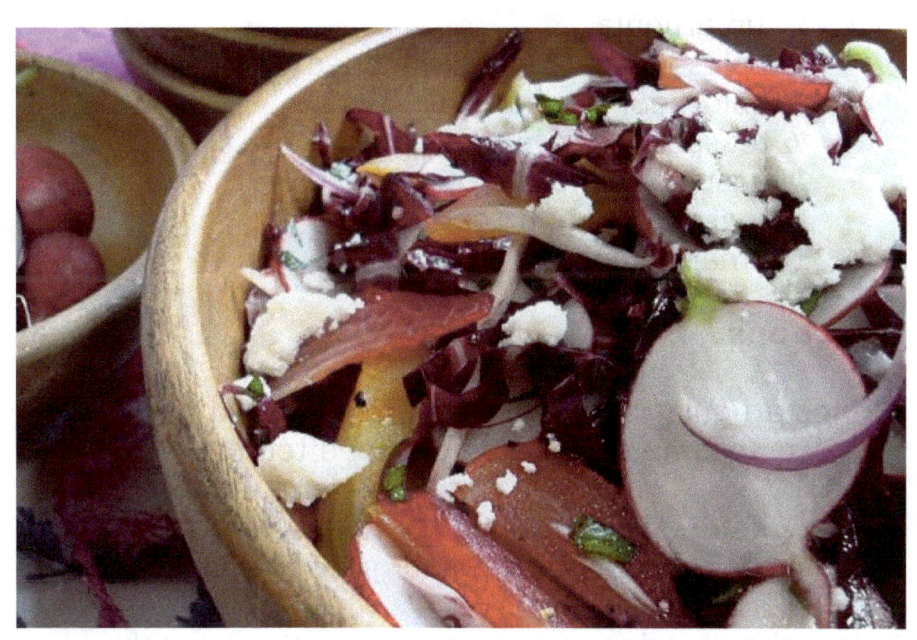

Green Salad with Walnuts

Prep Time:
10 minutes
Serve: 2

Ingredients:

- 1 cup arugula
- 2 tablespoons walnuts, chopped
- 1 tablespoon avocado oil
- ½ teaspoon sesame seeds
- 1 teaspoon lemon juice
- ½ teaspoon lemon zest, grated
- 1 tomato, chopped

Directions:

1.Chop arugula roughly and put in the salad bowl. Add walnuts, sesame seeds, and chopped tomato.

2.Make the dressing: mix up together avocado oil, sesame seeds, lemon juice, and grated lemon zest.

3.Pour the dressing over salad and shake it gently.

Nutrition: calories 71, fat 6, fiber 1.5, carbs 3.1, protein 2.7

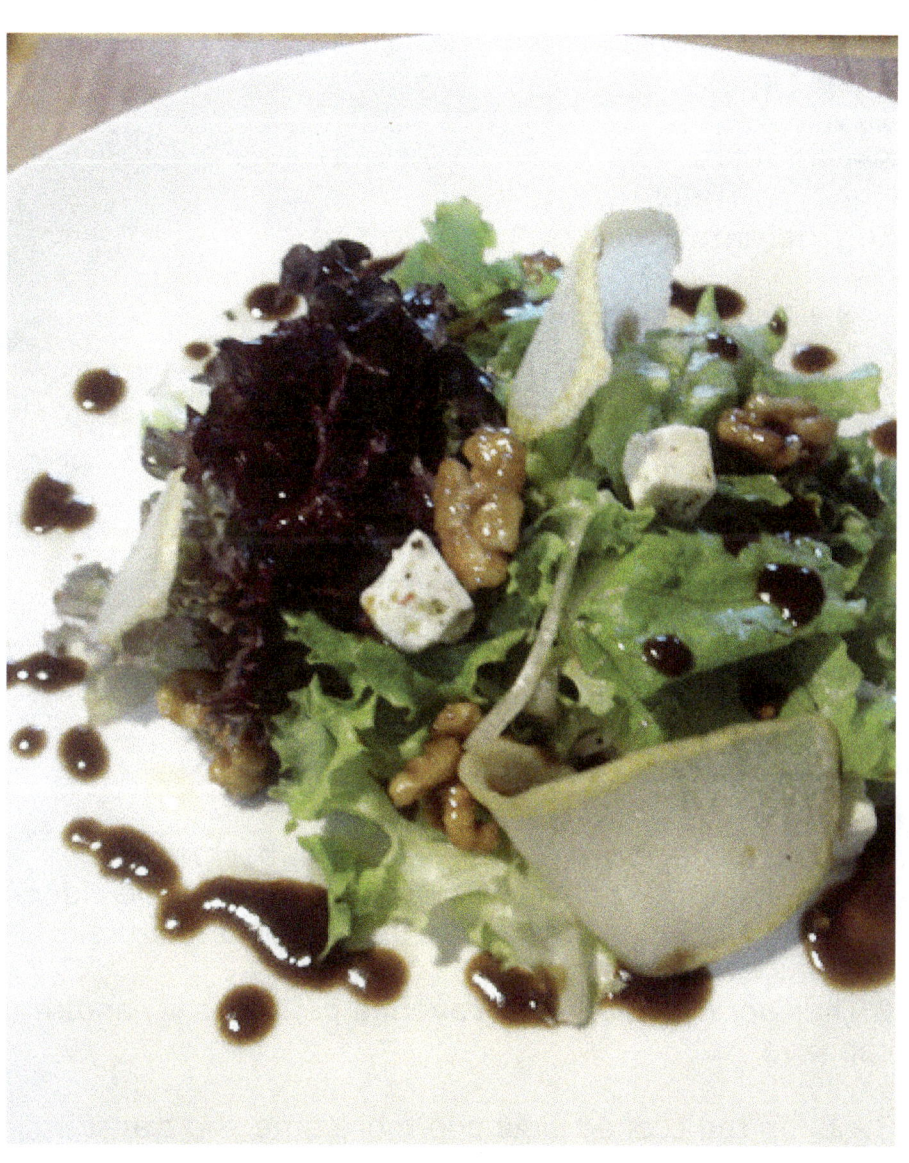

Jicama Slaw

Prep Time:
10 minutes
Serve: 4

Ingredients:

- 1 cup jicama, julienned
- 1 bell pepper, julienned
- 1 onion, sliced
- 1 tablespoon fresh cilantro, chopped
- ½ carrot, julienned
- 2 tablespoons olive oil
- 1 teaspoon apple cider vinegar
- ½ teaspoon cayenne pepper
- ½ teaspoon salt
- 1/3 cup red cabbage, shredded
- ¼ teaspoon liquid stevia

Directions:

1. In the mixing bowl, combine jicama, bell pepper, sliced onion, fresh cilantro, carrot, olive oil, apple cider vinegar, and liquid stevia. Mix up the salad mixture.

2. Then sprinkle slaw with cayenne pepper, salt, and red cabbage.

3. Mix up the cooked slaw one more time and transfer on the plates.

Nutrition: calories 98, fat 7.2, fiber 2.9, carbs 8.7, protein 1

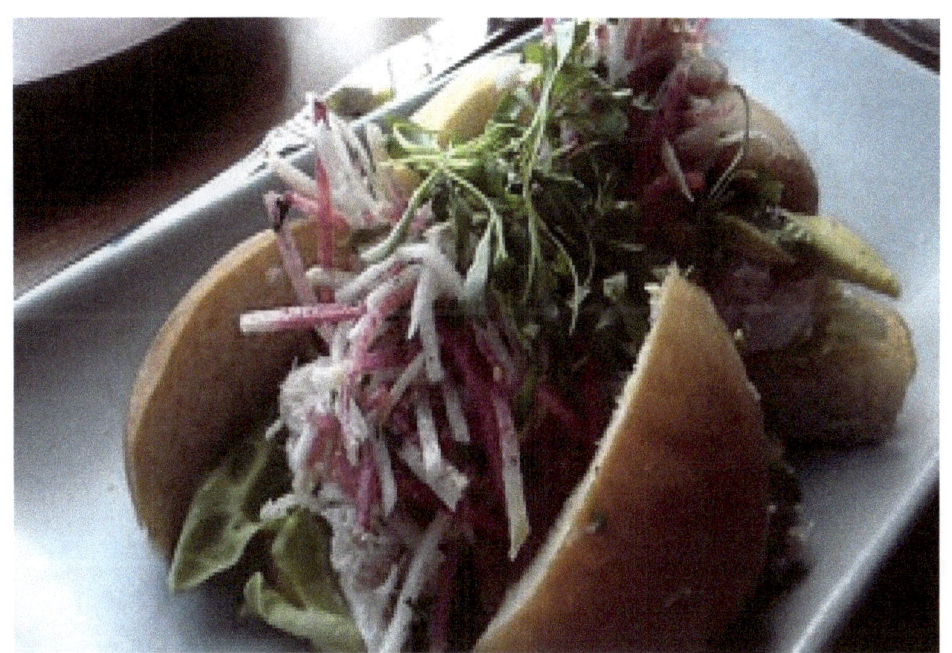

Peanut Slaw

Prep Time:
10 minutes
Serve: 4

Ingredients:

- 1 cup white cabbage
- 1 teaspoon peanut butter
- 1 teaspoon lemon juice
- 1 tablespoon peanuts, chopped
- ½ teaspoon ground black pepper
- 1 tablespoon canola oil
- 1 oz scallions, chopped
- 1 teaspoon sriracha
- ¼ cup fresh parsley, chopped

Directions:

1. Shred the white cabbage and transfer in the mixing bowl. Add peanuts, chopped fresh parsley, and scallions.

2. Then make the slaw dressing: whisk together peanut butter, lemon juice, ground black pepper, and canola oil.

3. Pour the dressing over the white cabbage mixture.

4. Add sriracha and chopped parsley.

5. Shake the slaw gently and transfer on the plates.

Nutrition: calories 62, fat 5.4, fiber 1.1, carbs 2.9, protein 1.4

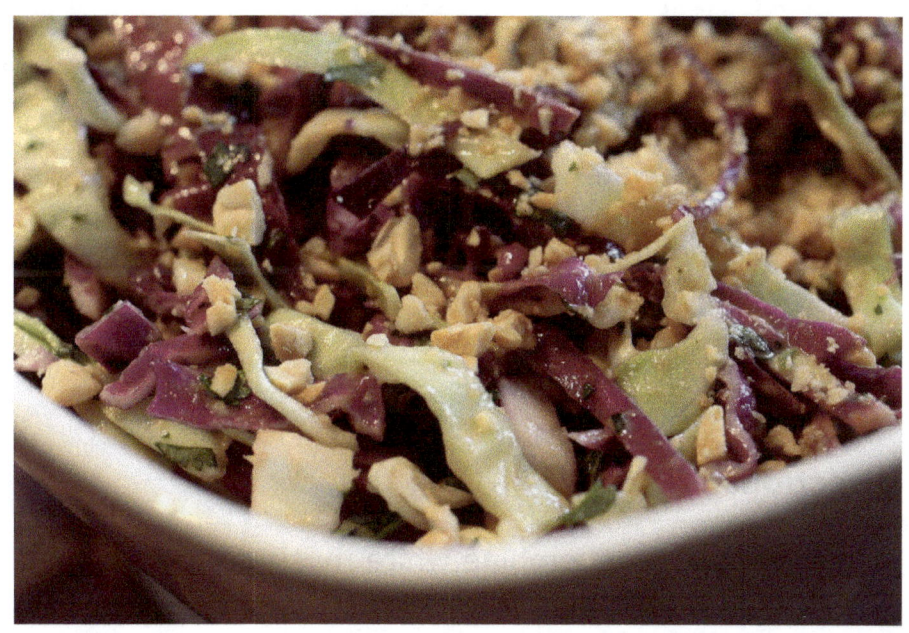

White Mushroom Saute

Prep Time:
15 minutes
Cook Time:
25 minutes
Serve: 6

Ingredients:

- 10 oz white mushrooms, chopped
- 1 carrot, chopped
- 1 onion, chopped
- ½ cup of water
- 3 tablespoons coconut cream
- 1 teaspoon salt
- ½ teaspoon turmeric
- 1 teaspoon chili flakes
- 1 teaspoon coconut oil
- ½ teaspoon Italian seasoning

Directions:

1. In the saucepan, combine white mushrooms, chopped carrot, onion, and mix up gently.

2. Sprinkle the vegetables with coconut cream, salt, turmeric, chili flakes, and coconut oil.

3. Add Italian seasoning and mix up well.

4. Cook the mixture over the high heat for 5 minutes.

5. Stir the vegetables constantly.

6. Then add water and close the lid.

7.Saute the meal for 20 minutes over the medium heat.

8.Then let saute rest for 10 minutes before.

Nutrition: calories 47, fat 2.9, fiber 1.3, carbs 4.9, protein 1.9

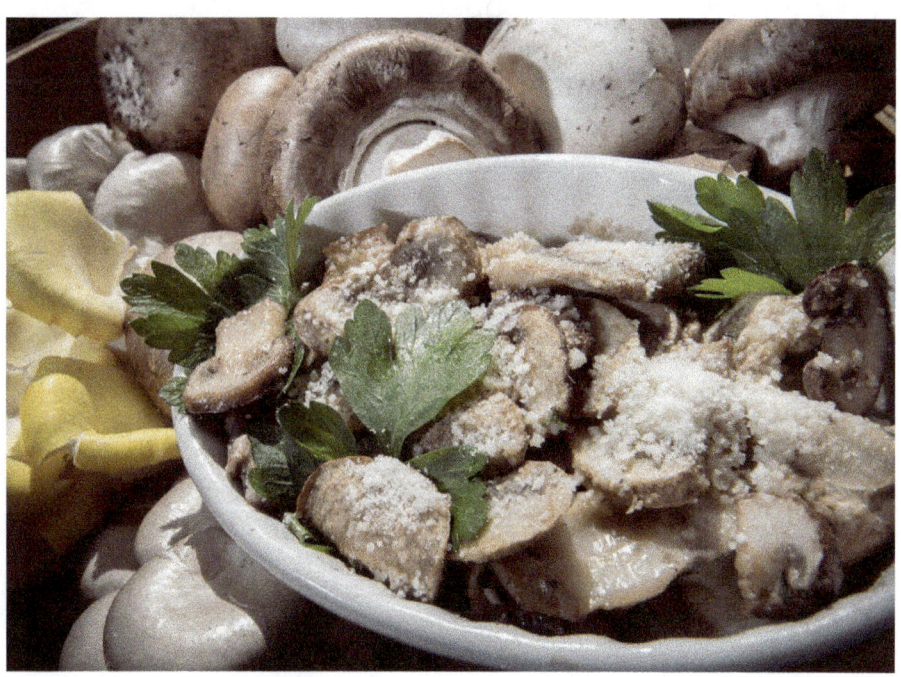

Caesar Salad

Prep Time:
15 minutes
Serve: 5

Ingredients:

- 1 tablespoon capers
- 2 cups lettuce, chopped
- 1 teaspoon walnuts, chopped
- 1 teaspoon mustard
- 2 tablespoons canola oil
- 1 teaspoon lime juice
- ½ teaspoon white pepper
- 1 avocado, peeled, chopped

Directions:

1. Place walnuts, mustard, canola oil, lime juice, white pepper, and avocado in the blender.

2. Blend the mixture until smooth.

3. After this, transfer the avocado smooth mixture in the salad bowl.

4. Add chopped lettuce.

5. Sprinkle the salad with capers. Don't stir the salad before.

Nutrition: calories 142, fat 14, fiber 3.1, carbs 4.6, protein 1.2

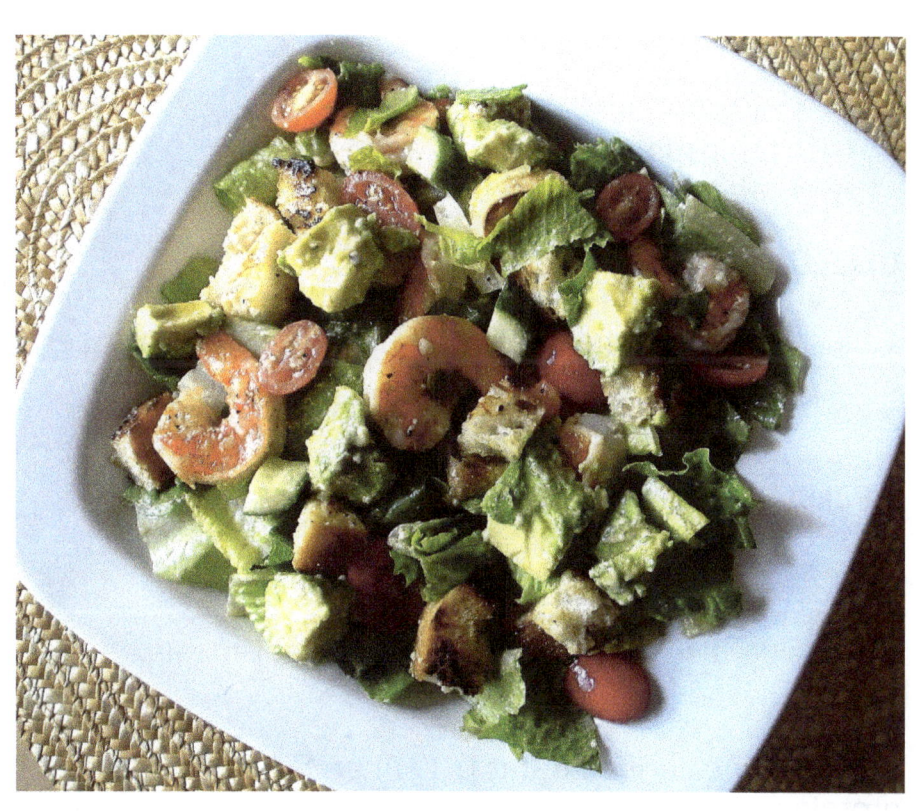

Cranberry Relish

Prep Time:
5 minutes
Serve: 6

Ingredients:

- 1 cup cranberries
- 1 orange, peeled, chopped
- 1 tablespoon Erythritol
- 3 tablespoons lemon juice

Directions:

1. Place cranberries and chopped orange in the blender.

2. Add Erythritol and lemon juice.

3. Pulse the ingredients for 1 minute.

4. Transfer the relish in the plate.

5. The side dish tastes the best with meat meals.

Nutrition: calories 26, fat 0.1, fiber 1.4 carbs 5.4, protein 0.4

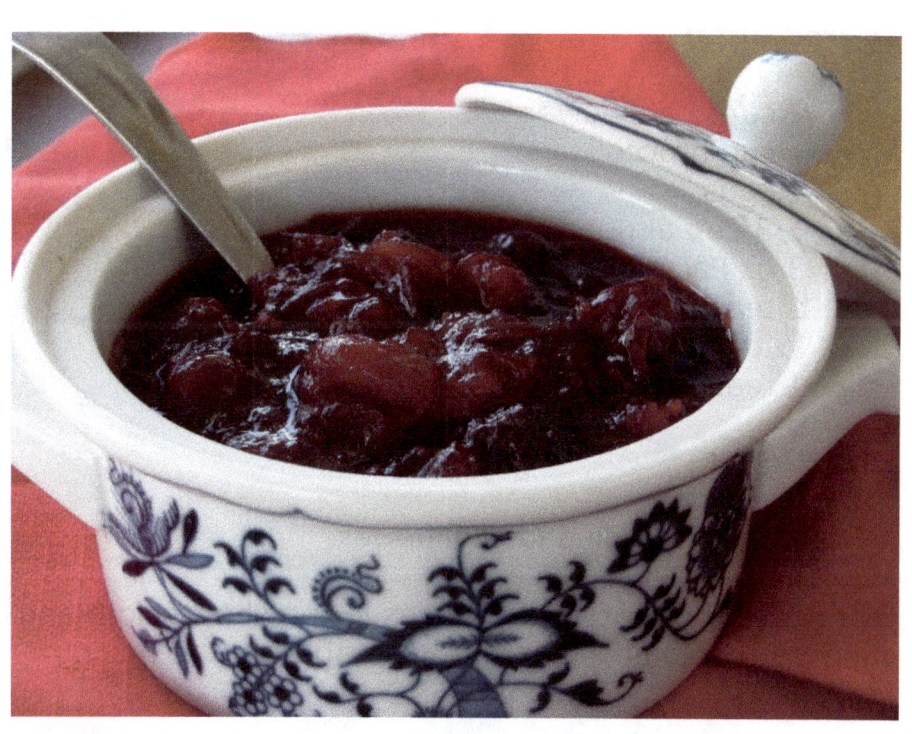

Vegetable Tots

Prep Time:
15 minutes
Cook Time:
12 minutes
Serve: 8

Ingredients:

- 2 cups cauliflower
- 1 cup broccoli
- 4 eggs
- 1/3 cup almond flour
- 3 oz Parmesan, grated
- 1 teaspoon ground coriander
- ½ teaspoon ground thyme
- 1 teaspoon olive oil

Directions:

1. Grate the broccoli and cauliflower.

2. Transfer the grated vegetables in the cheesecloth and squeeze the liquid. Then put vegetables in the mixing bowl.

3. Beat the eggs in the mixture and add grated cheese.

4. Then add almond flour, ground coriander, ground thyme, and mix it up.

5. Line the baking tray with baking paper and brush with 1 teaspoon of olive oil.

6.Make the medium size tots from the vegetable mixture and put them in the baking tray.

7.Bake the vegetable tots for 12 minutes at 365F.

8.Chill the meal to the room temperature before.

Nutrition: calories 88, fat 5.7, fiber 1.1, carbs 2.9, protein 7.3

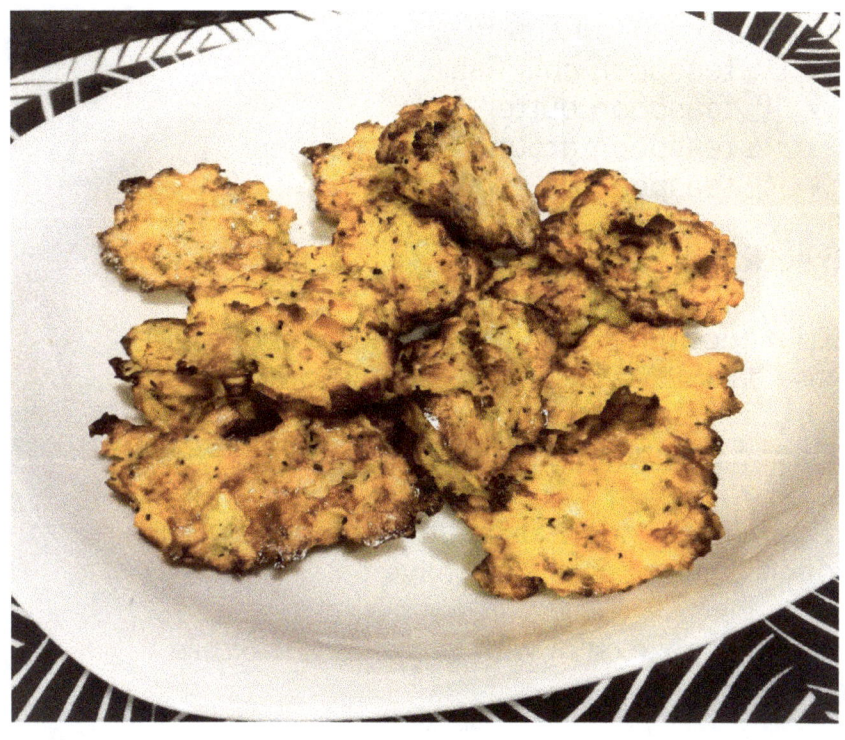

Hasselback Zucchini

Prep Time:
15 minutes
Cook Time:
20 minutes
Serve: 3

Ingredients:
- 3 small zucchini
- 4 oz Parmesan, sliced
- 1 tablespoon cream
- ½ teaspoon chili flakes
- ½ teaspoon butter
- ½ teaspoon ground black pepper
- ½ teaspoon olive oil

Directions:

1. Trim zucchini and cut them in the shape of the Hasselback.

2. Fill the zucchini Hasselback with sliced Parmesan.

3. Then whisk together cream, chili flakes, butter, ground black pepper, and olive oil.

4. Brush the zucchini with the cream mixture generously.

5. Wrap the zucchini Hasselback in the foil.

6. Preheat the oven to 365F.

7. Put the wrapped zucchini in the oven and cook for 20 minutes.

8. When the time is over, chill the zucchini for 5 minutes and then discard the foil.

9. Transfer the meal on the plates.

Nutrition: calories 156, fat 9.9, fiber 1.4, carbs 5.7, protein 13.7

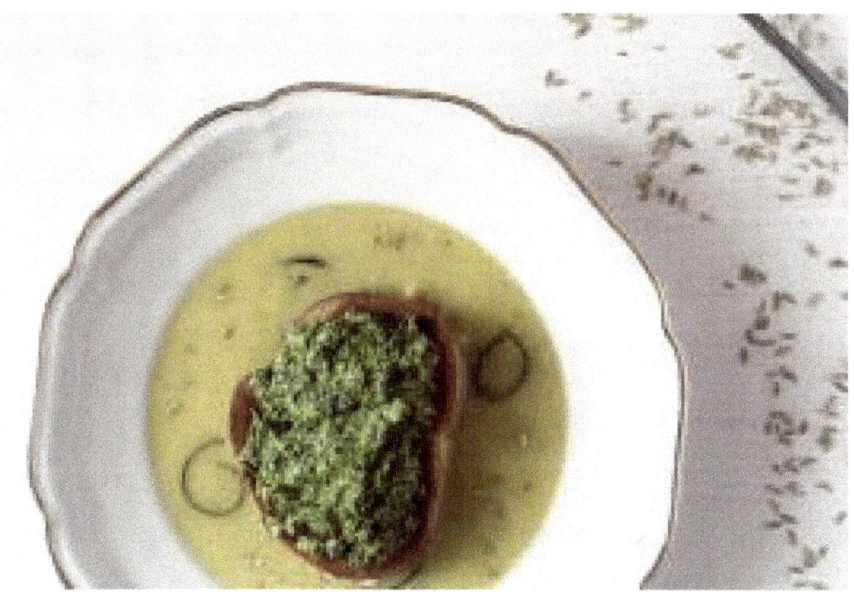

Lime Fennel Bulb

Prep Time:
10 minutes
Cook Time:
15 minutes
Serve: 4

Ingredients:

- 9 oz fennel bulb
- ½ lime
- 2 tablespoons butter
- 1 teaspoon olive oil
- 1 teaspoon harissa
- ½ teaspoon salt

Directions:

1. Cut every fennel bulb into 4 pieces.

2. Sprinkle the fennel with olive oil, harissa, and salt. Massage the fennel pieces with the help of the fingertips and transfer in the tray.

3. Add butter and bake fennel for 15 minutes at 360F. Stir the vegetables once during cooking.

Nutrition: calories 87, fat 7.3, fiber 2.2, carbs 6, protein 1

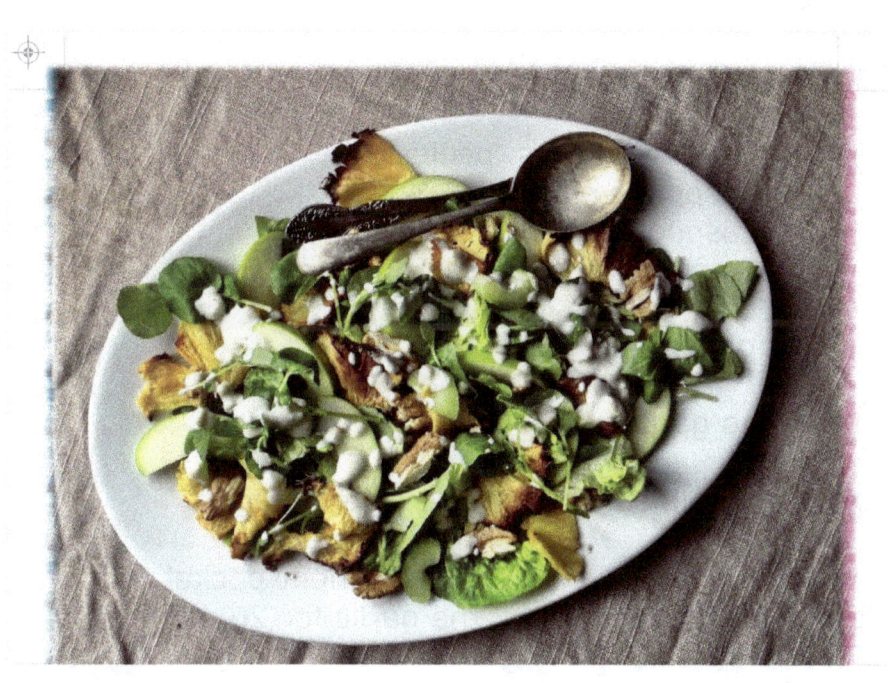

Baked Garlic

Prep Time:
5 minutes
Cook Time:
20 minutes
Serve: 3

Ingredients:

- 3 big garlic cloves, peeled
- 3 teaspoons olive oil
- 1 teaspoon salt
- ½ teaspoon apple cider vinegar

Directions:

1. Place the garlic cloves in the parchment.

2. Add olive oil, salt, and apple cider vinegar.

3. Wrap the garlic to get the parchment pocket and place it in the oven. Cook the garlic for 20 minutes at 355F.

4. When the time is over, the garlic should be very soft. Serve the garlic with all remaining gravy.

Nutrition: calories 54, fat 4.7, fiber 0.2, carbs 3, protein 0.6

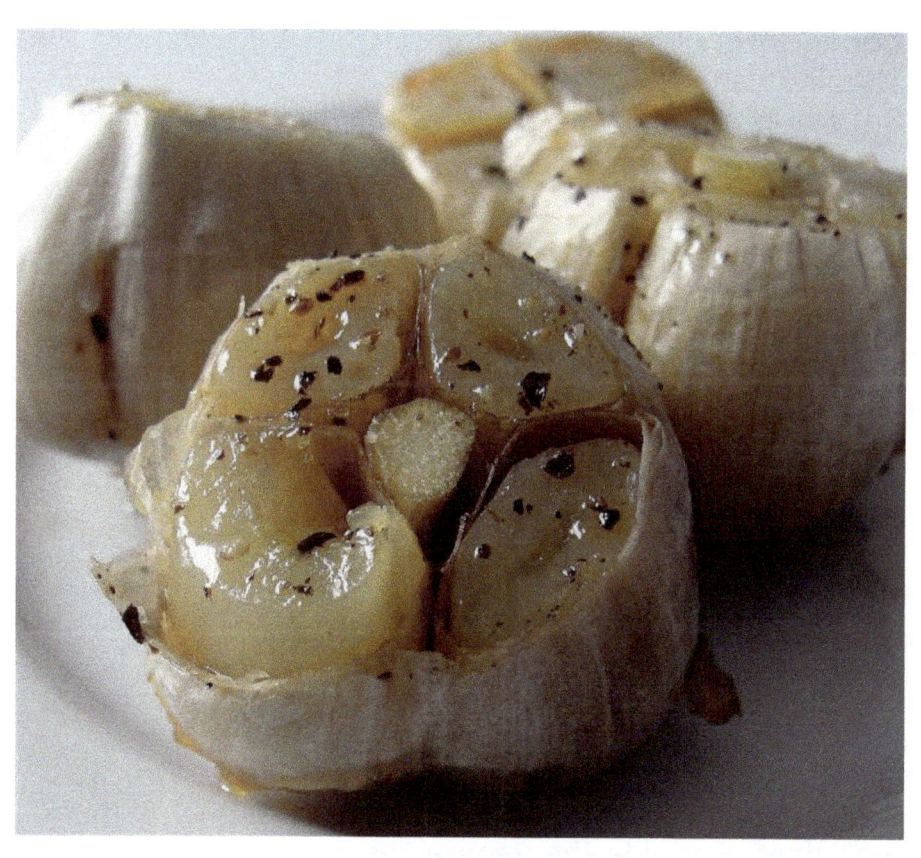

Roasted Okra

Prep Time:
10 minutes
Cook Time:
15 minutes
Serve: 4

Ingredients

- 1 ½ cup okra
- 1 tablespoon almond flour
- 1 teaspoon salt
- 1 tablespoon coconut oil
- ½ teaspoon cayenne pepper
- ½ teaspoon dried cilantro
- 1 tablespoon heavy cream

Directions:

1. Slice the okra roughly.

2. Put coconut oil in the skillet.

3. Add sliced okra and start to cook it over the medium-high heat. Sprinkle the vegetables with salt, cayenne pepper, and dried cilantro. Then add heavy cream and mix up well.

4. Cook okra for 5 minutes more.

5. Sprinkle the vegetables with almond flour and close the lid.

6.Cook the side dish for 5 minutes over the medium heat.

Nutrition: calories 98, fat 8.4, fiber 2, carbs 4.5, protein 2.3

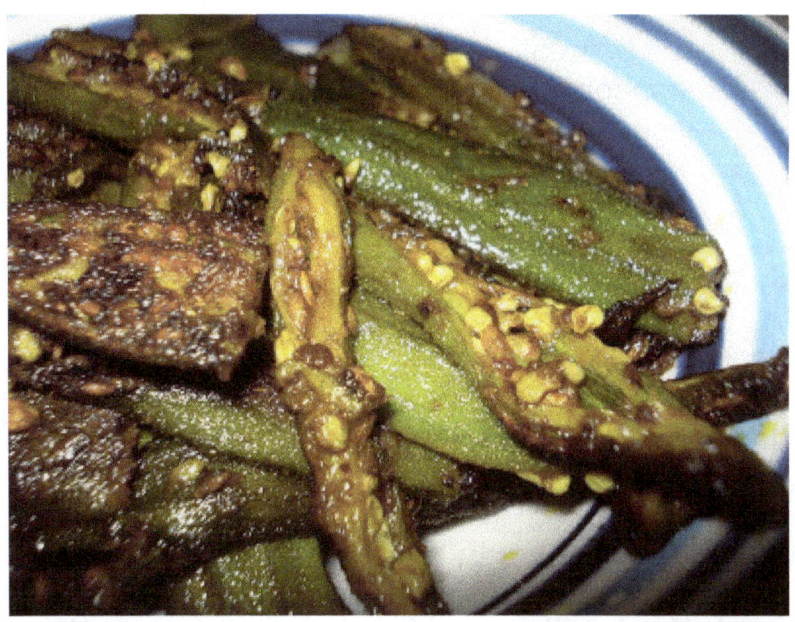

Broccoli Gratin

Prep Time:
10 minutes
Cook Time:
30 minutes
Serve: 6

Ingredients:

- 2 cups broccoli florets
- 1 teaspoon salt
- 1 teaspoon chili flakes
- 3 eggs, whisked
- 2 oz Swiss cheese, grated
- 1 onion, diced
- 1 cup heavy cream

Directions:

1. Whisk together chili flakes, salt, eggs, and heavy cream.

2. Add the diced onion in the mixture and stir gently.

3. After this, place broccoli florets into the non-sticky gratin mold.

4. Sprinkle the vegetables with Swiss cheese and heavy cream mixture.

5. Cover the gratin with foil and secure the edges.

6. Cook gratin for 30 minutes in the preheated to the 360F oven.

7. When the time is over, discard the foil and check if the broccoli is tender.

8. Chill the gratin little and transfer on the plates.

Nutrition: calories 154, fat 12.3, fiber 1.2, carbs 5, protein 6.8

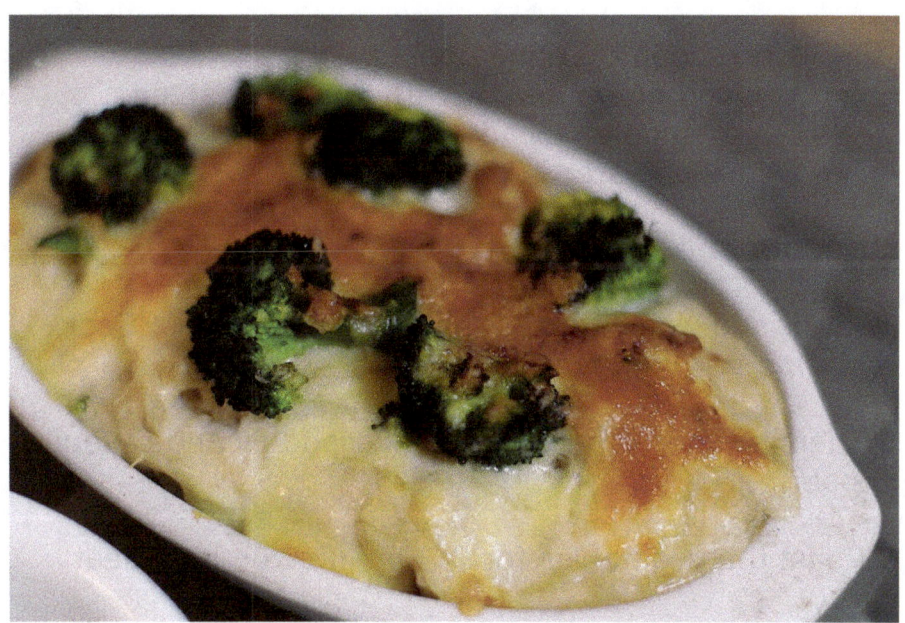

Cayenne Pepper Green Beans

Prep Time:
10 minutes
Cook Time:
20 minutes
Serve: 4

Ingredients:

- 1 teaspoon cayenne pepper
- 1 pound green beans, trimmed and halved
- 1 tablespoon avocado oil
- 2 cups of water

Directions:

1. Bring the water to boil and add green beans. Cook them for 10 minutes.

2. Then remove water and add avocado oil and cayenne pepper.

3. Roast the vegetables for 2-3 minutes on high heat.

Nutrition: 41 calories, 2.2g protein, 8.5g carbohydrates, 0.7g fat, 4.1g fiber, 0mg cholesterol, 11mg sodium, 258mg potassium.

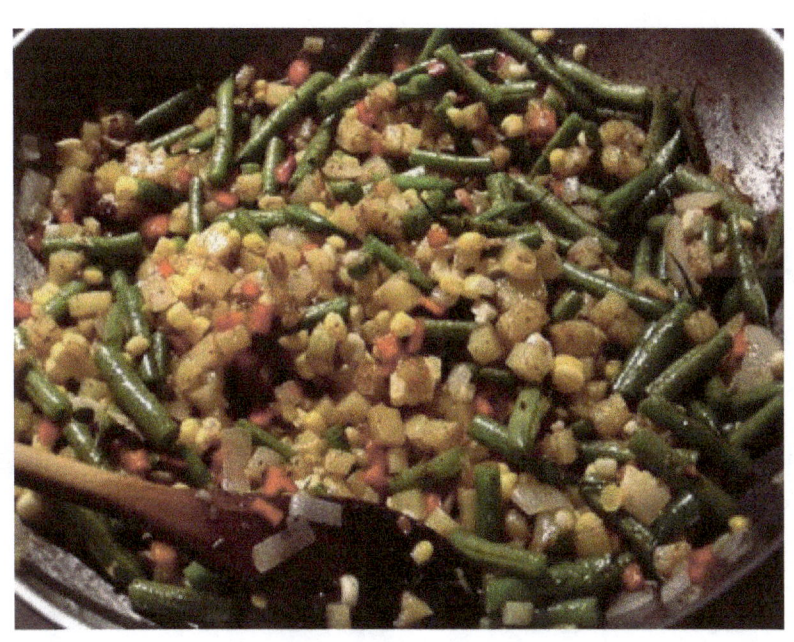

Lime Brussels Sprouts

Prep Time:
10 minutes
Cook Time:
20 minutes
Serve: 4

Ingredients:

- 2 pounds Brussels sprouts, trimmed and halved
- 1 tablespoon olive oil
- 2 tablespoons lime juice
- 1 teaspoon lime zest, grated
- 1 teaspoon ground paprika

Directions:

1. Mix Brussel sprouts with olive oil, lime juice, lime zest, and ground paprika.

2. Put the vegetables in the lined with the baking paper tray and bake for 20 minutes at 365F.

Nutrition: 130 calories, 7.8g protein, 21g carbohydrates, 4.3g fat, 8.8g fiber, 0mg cholesterol, 57mg sodium, 895mg potassium.

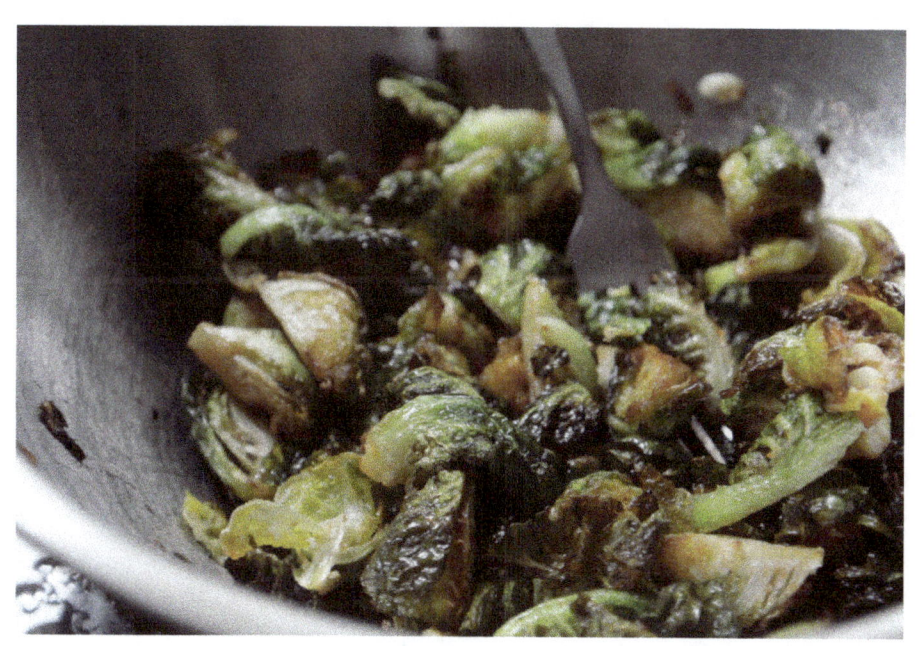

Cabbage Bowl

Prep Time:
10 minutes
Cook Time:
20 minutes
Serve: 4

Ingredients:

- 4 cups white cabbage
- 1 cup tomatoes, diced
- 2 tablespoons olive oil
- 2 cups of water
- 1 teaspoon dried parsley

Directions:

1. Mix white cabbage with tomatoes in the saucepan.

2. Add water, dried parsley, and olive oil.

3. Close the lid and simmer the meal on medium heat for 20 minutes.

Nutrition: 86 calories, 1.3g protein, 5.8g carbohydrates, 7.2g fat, 2.3g fiber, 0mg cholesterol, 19mg sodium, 229mg potassium.

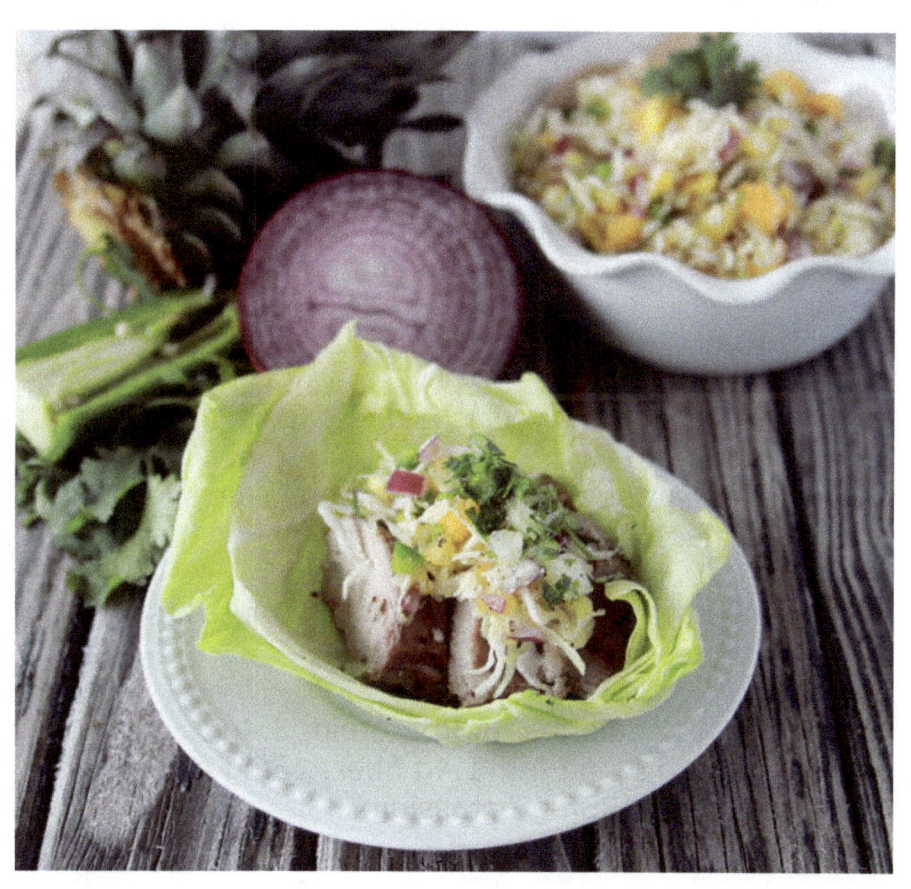

Parmesan Asparagus

Prep Time:
10 minutes
Cook Time:
15 minutes
Serve: 4

Ingredients:

- 3 oz Parmesan, grated
- 2 tablespoons olive oil
- 1 bunch asparagus, trimmed and halved

Directions:

1. Line the baking tray with baking paper.

2. Put the asparagus in the tray in one layer and sprinkle it with Parmesan and olive oil.

3. Bake the asparagus at 385F for 15 minutes.

Nutrition: 142 calories, 8.3g protein, 3.4g carbohydrates, 11.6g fat, 1.4g fiber, 15mg cholesterol, 199mg sodium, 135mg potassium.

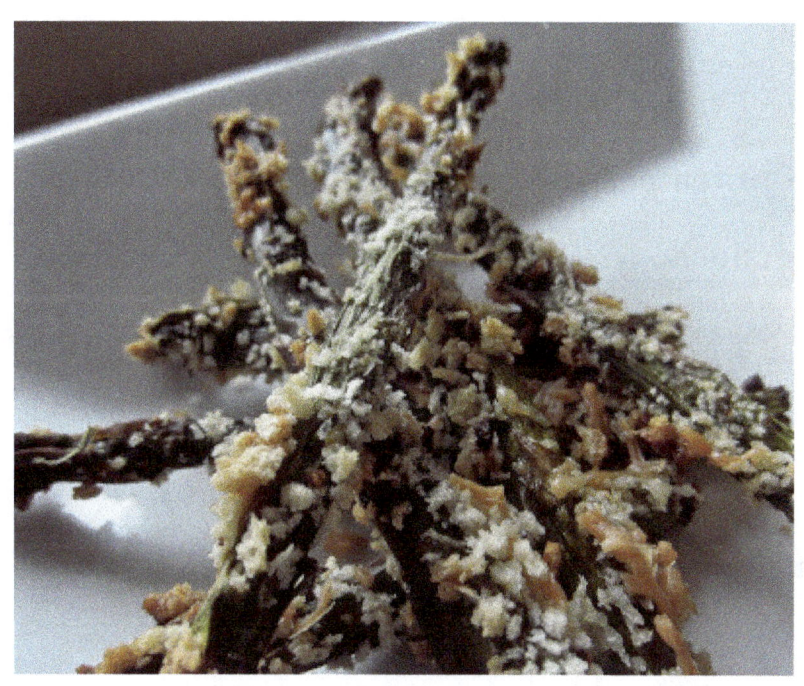

Coconut Quinoa

Prep Time:
10 minutes
Cook Time:
25 minutes
Serve: 4

Ingredients:

- 1 cup quinoa
- 2 cups of water
- 1 cup of coconut milk
- 1 teaspoon ground turmeric

Directions:

1. Mix water with quinoa and coconut milk.

2. Add ground turmeric and close cook the meal on low heat for 25 minutes.

Nutrition: 296 calories, 7.4g protein, 31g carbohydrates, 16.9g fat, 4.4g fiber, 0mg cholesterol, 15mg sodium, 412mg potassium.

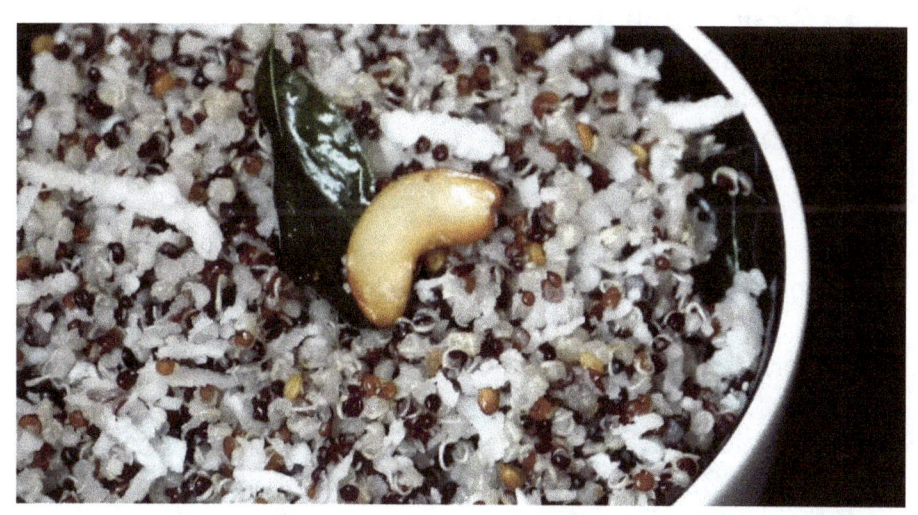

Rosemary Black Beans

Prep Time:
10 minutes
Cook Time:
0 minutes
Serve: 4

Ingredients:

- 1 tablespoon avocado oil
- 2 cups canned black beans, drained and rinsed
- 1 tablespoon dried rosemary
- 1 tablespoon lemon juice
- 1 onion, sliced

Directions:

1. Mix black beans with dried rosemary and lemon juice.

2. Add onion and avocado oil. Shake the meal well.

Nutrition: 350 calories, 21.4g protein, 63.9g carbohydrates, 2g fat, 15.9g fiber, 0mg cholesterol, 7mg sodium, 1502mg potassium.

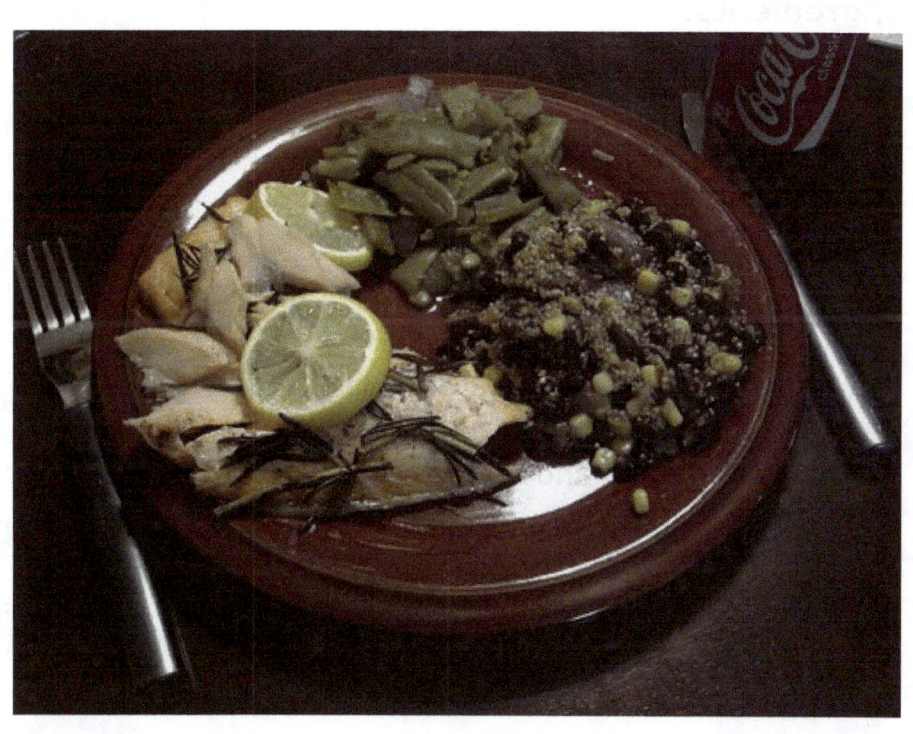

Oregano Green Beans

Prep Time:
10 minutes
Cook Time:
15 minutes
Serve: 4

Ingredients:

- 1 pound green beans, trimmed and halved
- 1 cup of water
- 1 tablespoon dried oregano
- 1 teaspoon chili powder
- 1 tablespoon almond butter

Directions:

1. Bring the water to boil.

2. Add green beans and boil them for 10 minutes.

3. Then transfer the green beans in the bowl and add dried oregano, chili powder, and almond butter.

4. Stir the meal well.

Nutrition: 65 calories, 3.1g protein, 9.9g carbohydrates, 2.6g fat, 5g fiber, 0mg cholesterol, 16mg sodium, 299mg potassium.

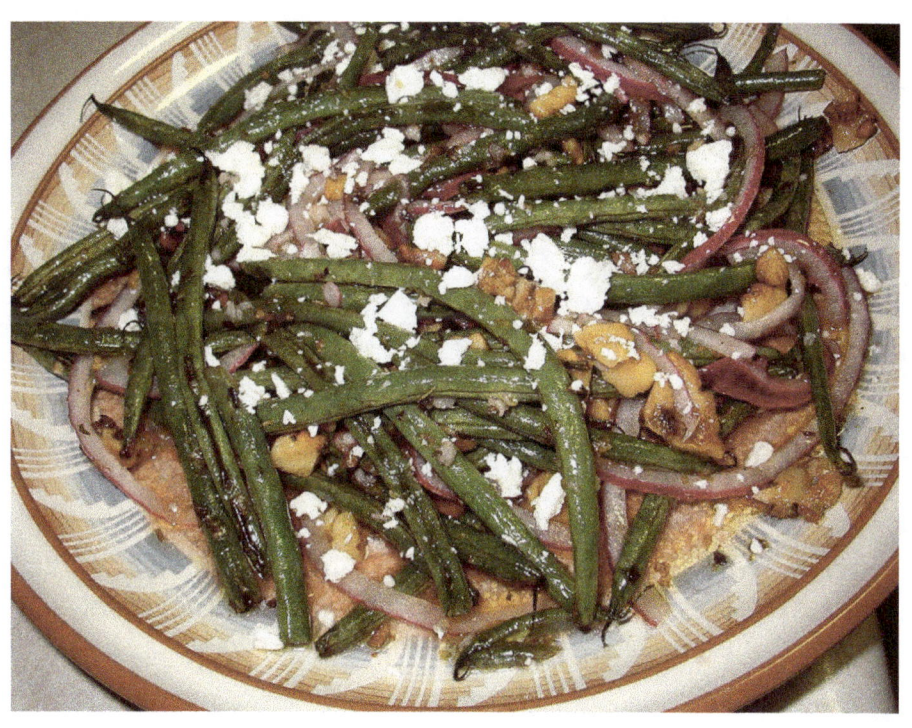

Yam Mash

Prep Time:
10 minutes
Cook Time:
25 minutes
Serve: 4

Ingredients:

- 1-pound yams, peeled
- ¼ cup coconut cream
- 1 tablespoon dried dill

Directions:

1. Bake the yams at 365F for 25 minutes.

2. Then mash the yams and mix them with coconut cream and dried dill. Stir the meal well.

Nutrition: 168 calories, 2.2g protein, 32.4g carbohydrates, 3.8g fat, 4.9g fiber, 0mg cholesterol, 13mg sodium, 825mg potassium.

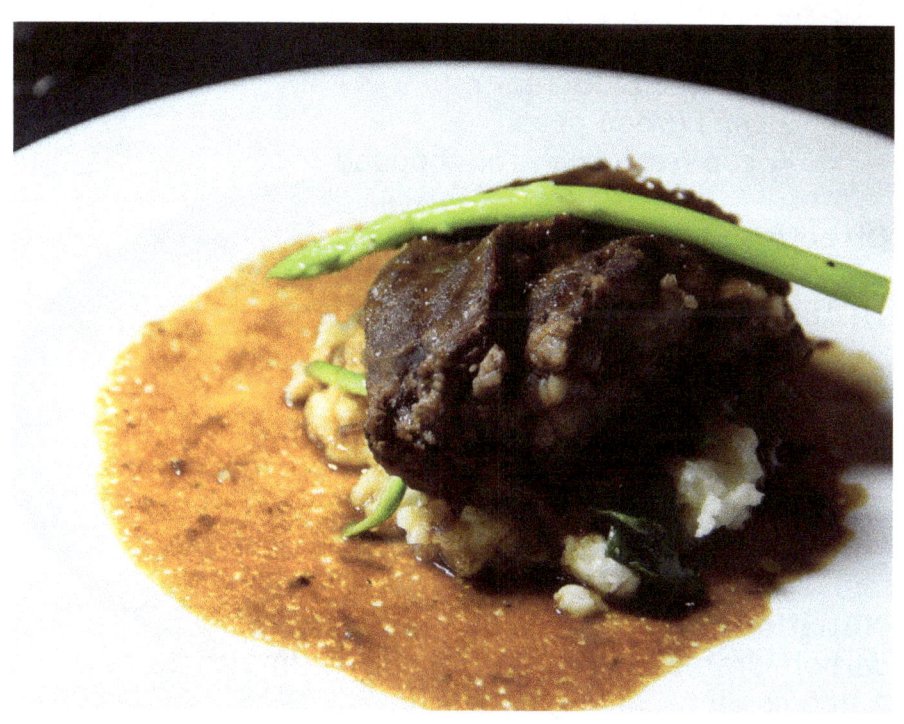

Soft Peas

Prep Time:
10 minutes
Cook Time:
20 minutes
Serve: 4

Ingredients:

- 1 cup coconut cream
- 2 cups green peas
- ¼ cup fresh cilantro, chopped

Directions:

1. Pour coconut cream in the saucepan.

2. Add green peas and cilantro.

3. Close the lid and cook the meal on medium heat for 20 minutes.

Nutrition: 197 calories, 5.3g protein, 13.8g carbohydrates, 14.6g fat, 5.1g fiber, 0mg cholesterol, 13mg sodium, 340mg potassium.

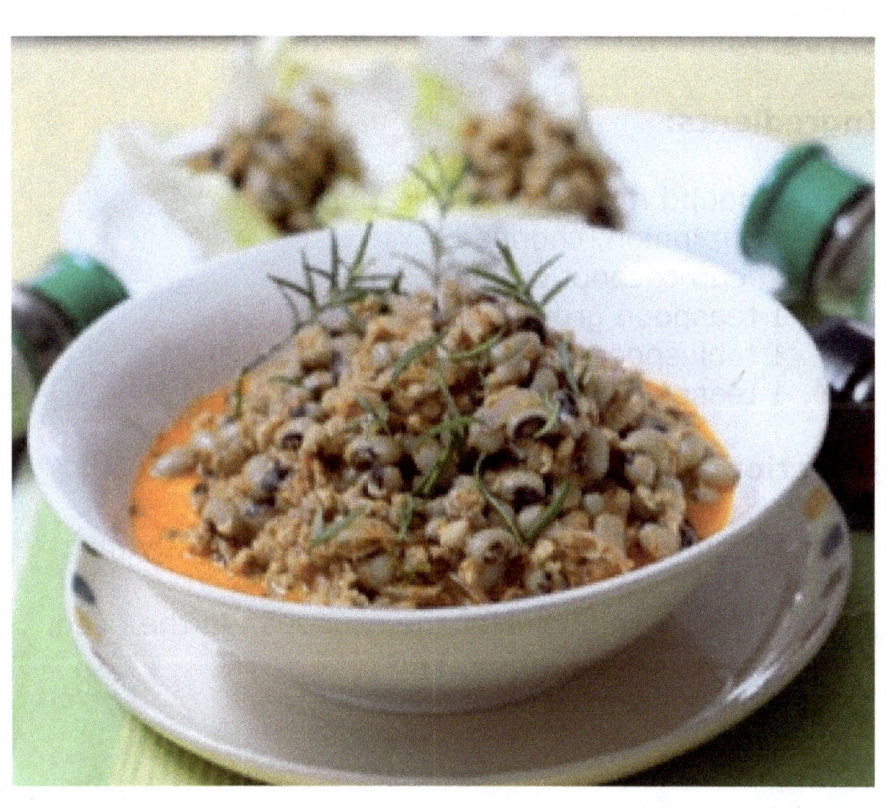

Mushroom Stew

Prep Time:
10 minutes
Cook Time:
35 minutes
Serve: 4

Ingredients:

- 1 pound mushrooms, sliced
- 1 cup onion, chopped
- ½ cup coconut cream
- 1 teaspoon ground black pepper
- 1 tablespoon olive oil
- 1 teaspoon dried dill

Directions:

1. Put all ingredients in the saucepan and gently mix.

2. Close the lid and transfer the saucepan in the oven.

3. Cook the stew at 365F for 35 minutes.

Nutrition: 137 calories, 4.7g protein, 8.6g carbohydrates, 1g fat, 2.6g fiber, 0mg cholesterol, 13mg sodium, 496mg potassium.

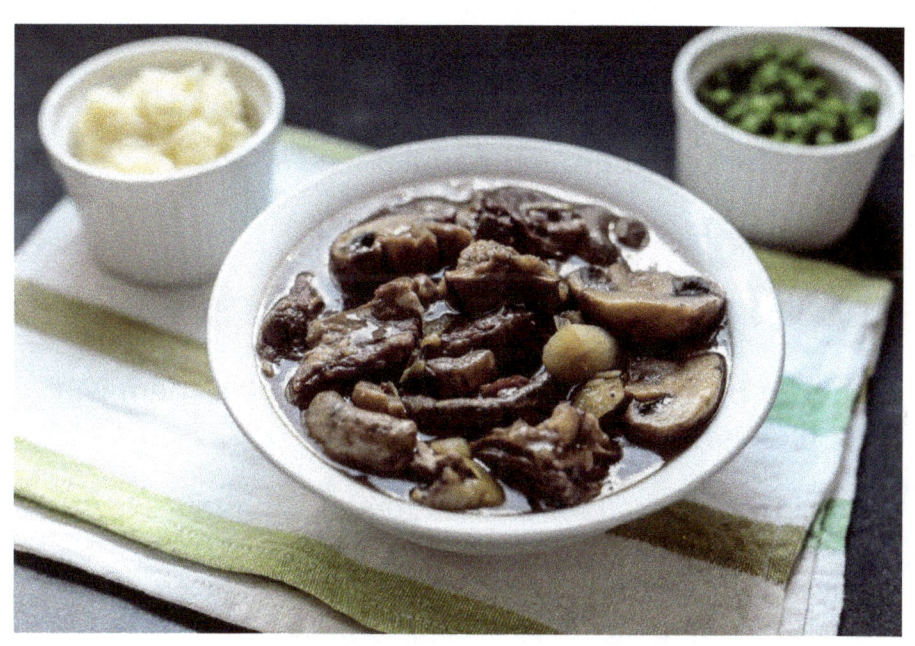

Cheesy Broccoli

Prep Time:
10 minutes
Cook Time:
25 minutes
Serve: 4

Ingredients:

- 1 pound broccoli florets
- 3 oz Romano cheese, grated
- 1 tablespoon olive oil
- ½ teaspoon ground paprika

Directions:

1. Line the baking tray with baking paper.

2. Put the broccoli florets inside and sprinkle them with olive oil and ground paprika.

3. Cook the broccoli for 20 minutes at 365F.

4. Then top the vegetables with Romano cheese and bake for 5 minutes more.

Nutrition: 152 calories, 10g protein, 8.4g carbohydrates, 9.6g fat, 3.1g fiber, 22mg cholesterol, 293mg sodium, 383mg potassium.

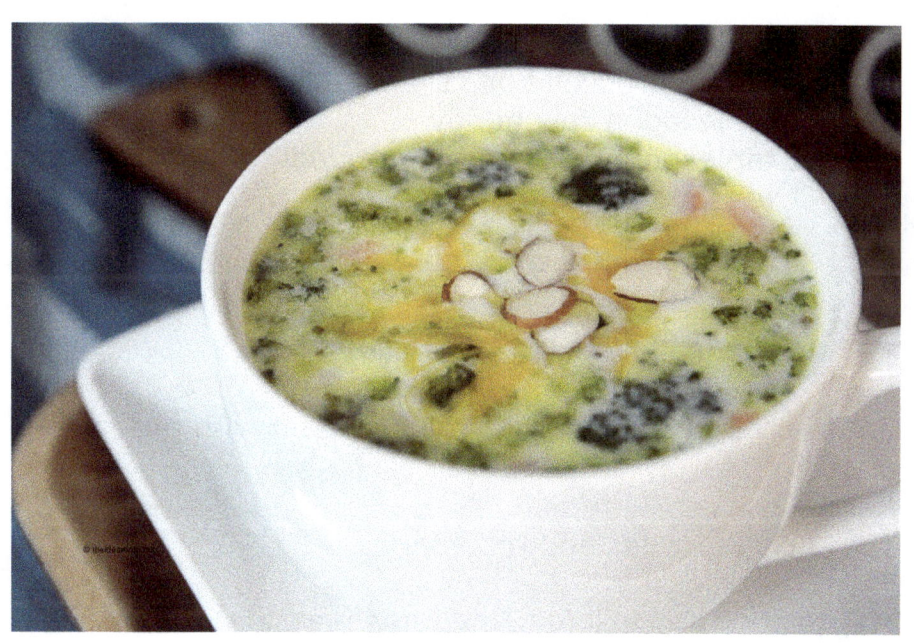

Glazed Broccoli

Prep Time:
10 minutes
Cook Time:
20 minutes
Serve: 4

Ingredients:

- 1 tablespoon avocado oil
- 1 pound broccoli florets
- 1 tablespoon raw honey
- 1 tablespoon rosemary, chopped
- 1 teaspoon chili powder

Directions:

1. Preheat the skillet well.

2. Add broccoli florets and sprinkle them with avocado oil.

3. Add chili powder and rosemary.

4. Roast the broccoli for 7 minutes per side.

5. Then add honey, carefully mix the vegetables and cook them for 3 minutes more.

Nutrition: 64 calories, 3.4g protein, 13g carbohydrates, 1.1g fat, 3.7g fiber, 0mg cholesterol, 45mg sodium, 393mg potassium.

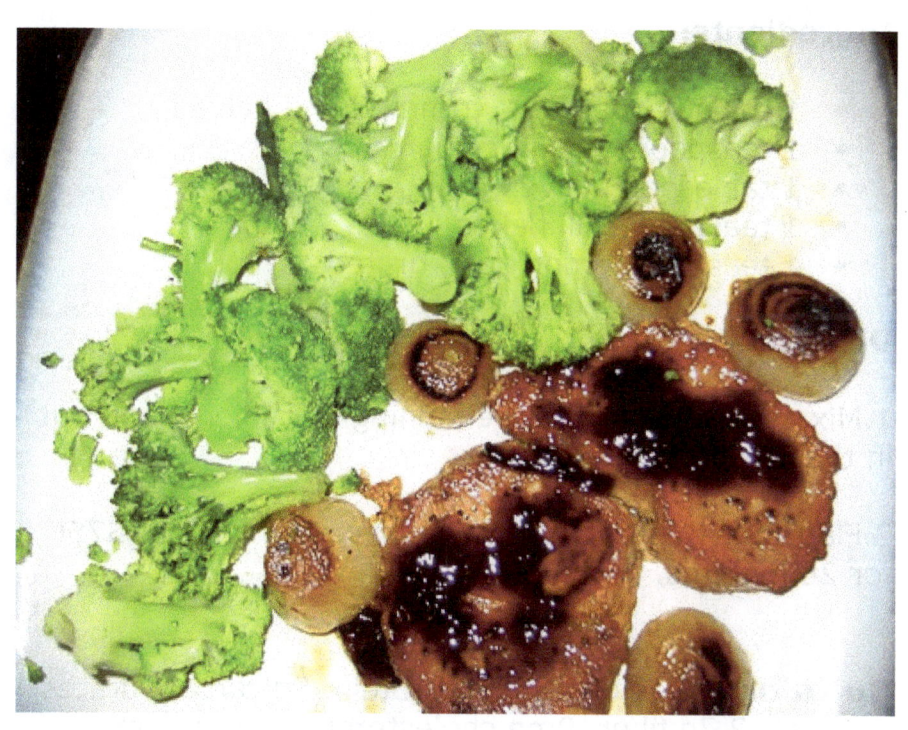

Cinnamon Asparagus

Prep Time:
10 minutes
Cook Time:
20 minutes
Serve: 4

Ingredients:

- 1 pound asparagus, trimmed and halved
- 1 teaspoon ground cinnamon
- 1 tablespoon olive oil
- 1 teaspoon chili flakes
- 1 teaspoon lemon zest, grated

Directions:

1. Mix asparagus with all remaining ingredients and put in the baking tray.

2. Flatten the asparagus in one layer and bake at 375F for 20 minutes.

Nutrition: 55 calories, 2.5g protein, 5g carbohydrates, 3.7g fat, 2.7g fiber, 0mg cholesterol, 2mg sodium, 234mg potassium.

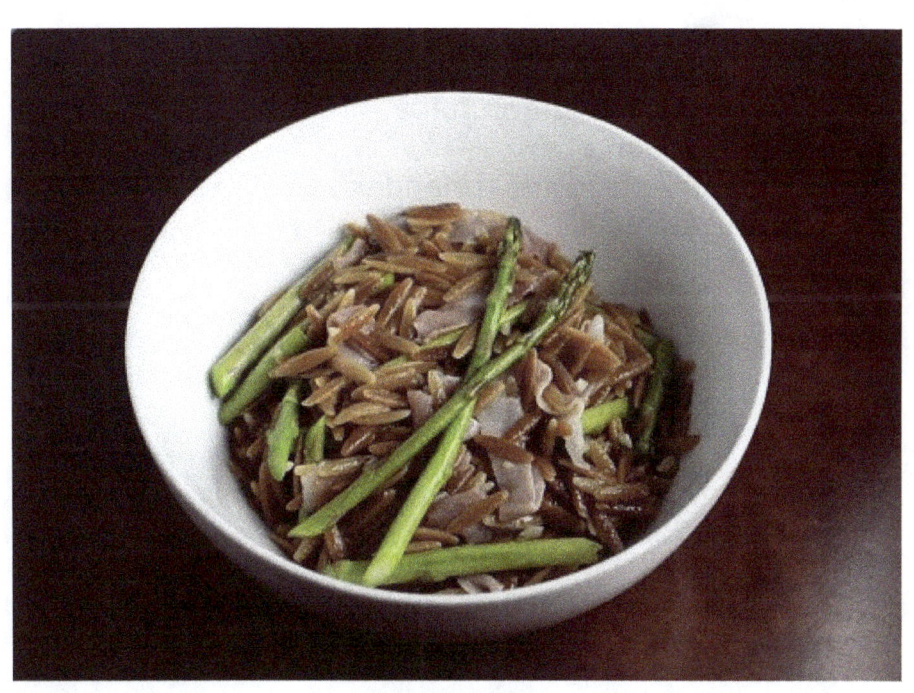

Spicy Cucumbers

Prep Time:
15 minutes
Cook Time:
0 minutes
Serve: 4

Ingredients:

- 3 cups cucumbers, chopped
- 3 tablespoons lemon juice
- 1 tablespoon olive oil
- 1 teaspoon ground coriander
- 1 teaspoon chili powder
- 1 teaspoon dried parsley

Directions:

1. Put the cucumbers in the big glass jar.

2. Add all remaining ingredients and carefully mix the mixture.

3. Leave it for at least 10 minutes to marinate.

Nutrition: 47 calories, 0.7g protein, 3.5g carbohydrates, 3.8g fat, 0.7g fiber, 0mg cholesterol, 11mg sodium, 143mg potassium.

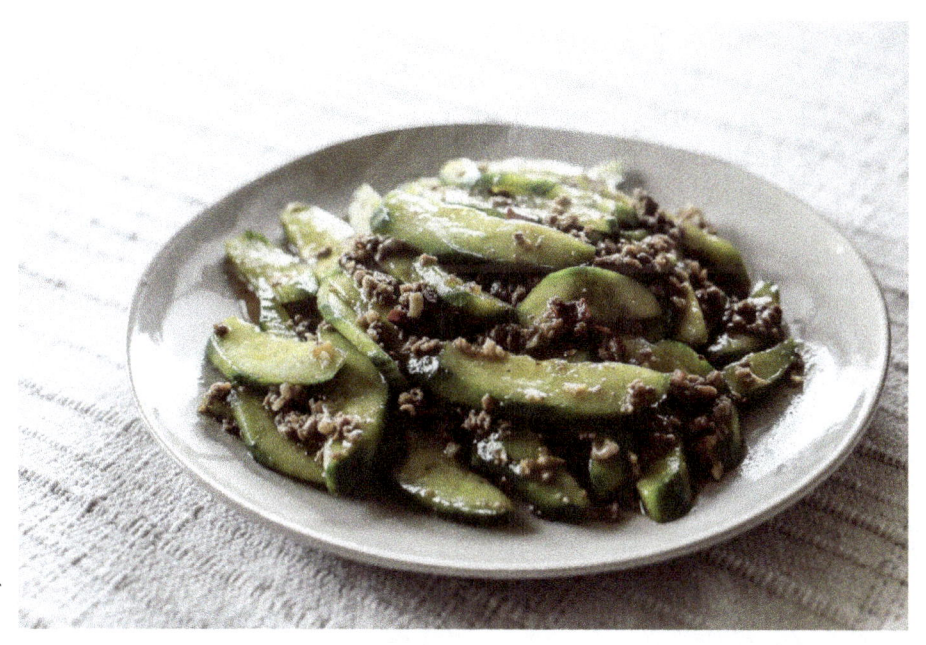

Summer Salad

Prep Time:
10 minutes
Cook Time:
0 minutes
Serve: 4

Ingredients:

- 1 pound cherry tomatoes, halved
- 2 sweet peppers, chopped
- 1 cucumber, chopped
- 2 tablespoons olive oil
- 2 garlic cloves, diced

Directions:

1.Mix cherry tomatoes with sweet peppers, cucumber, and garlic cloves.

2.Add olive oil and mix the salad well.

Nutrition: 113 calories, 2.2g protein, 12.1g carbohydrates, 7.5g fat, 2.6g fiber, 0mg cholesterol, 9mg sodium, 497mg potassium.

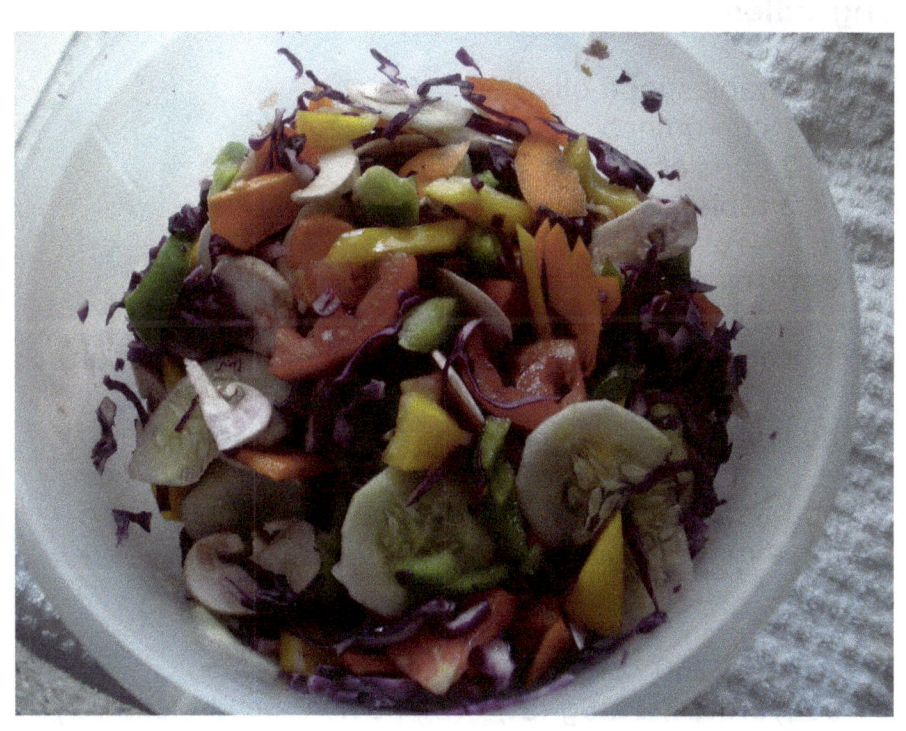

Tender Quinoa

Prep Time:
10 minutes
Cook Time:
30 minutes
Serve: 4

Ingredients:

- 1 tablespoon olive oil
- 1 cup quinoa
- 2 cups of water
- 3 tablespoons almond butter

Directions:

1. Mix quinoa with olive oil and put it in the saucepan.

2. Add water and boil it for 25 minutes on low heat.

3. Then add almond butter and cook the quinoa for 5 minutes more.

Nutrition: 260 calories, 8.6g protein, 29.5g carbohydrates, 12.8g fat, 4.2g fiber, 0mg cholesterol, 7mg sodium, 330mg potassium.

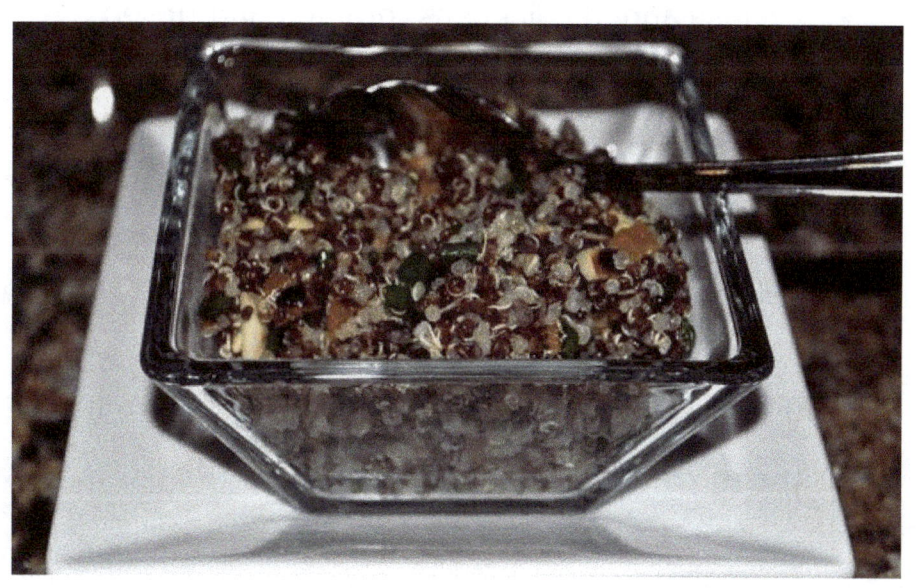

Chickpeas Bowl

Prep Time:
5 minutes
Cook Time:
0 minutes
Serve: 4

Ingredients:

- 2 cups canned chickpeas, drained and rinsed
- 1 tomato, chopped
- 1 cup fresh cilantro, chopped
- 1 tablespoon olive oil
- 2 garlic cloves, sliced
- 2 tablespoons lemon juice

Directions:

1. Mix chickpeas with tomatoes, cilantro, olive oil, garlic, and lemon juice.

2. Stir the mixture well and divide into serving bowls.

Nutrition: 402 calories, 19.7g protein, 62.1g carbohydrates, 9.7g fat, 17.8g fiber, 0mg cholesterol, 28mg sodium, 948mg potassium.

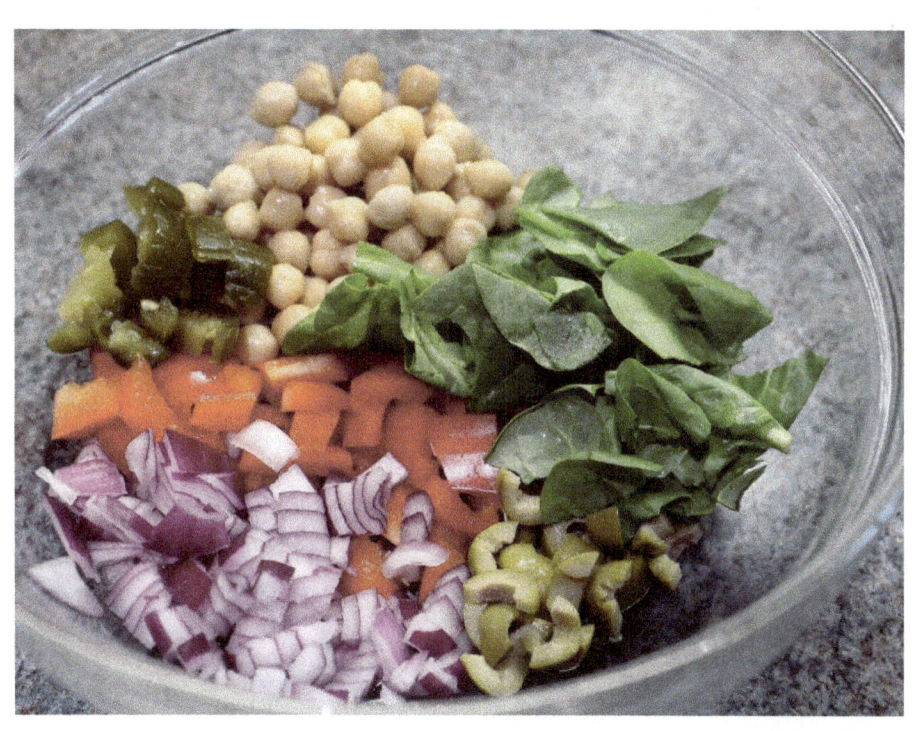

Beans Mash

Prep Time:
10 minutes
Cook Time:
0 minutes
Serve: 4

Ingredients:

- 16 oz white beans, boiled
- 1 tablespoon almond butter
- ¼ cup coconut cream
- ½ teaspoon ground clove

Directions:

1. Put the white beans in the blender.

2. Add almond butter, coconut cream, and ground clove.

3. Blend the mixture until smooth and transfer into the serving bowls.

Nutrition: 437 calories, 27.7g protein, 70.1g carbohydrates, 6.8g fat, 18.1g fiber, mg cholesterol, 21mg sodium, 2108mg potassium.

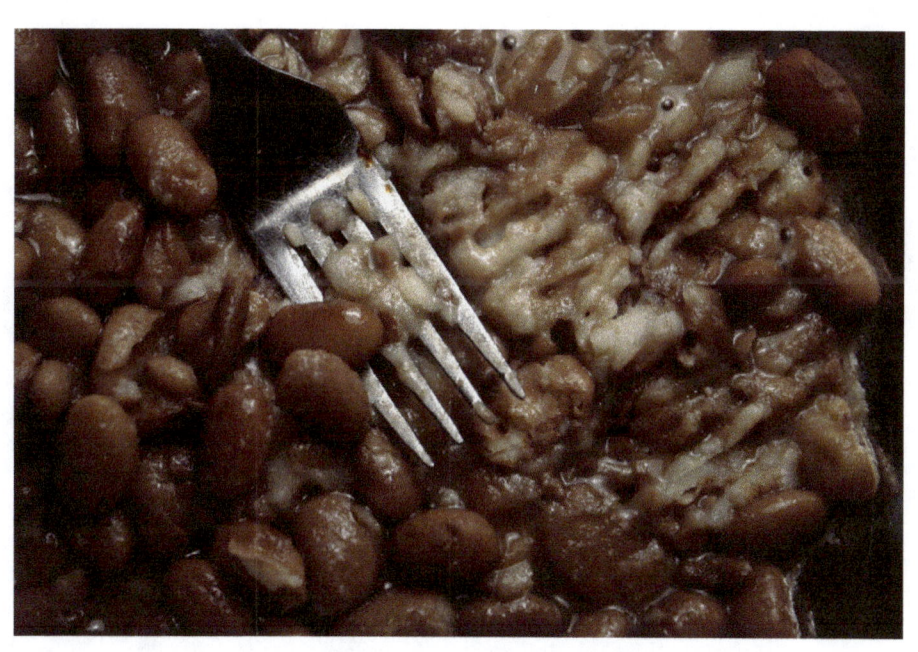

Spiralized Carrot

Prep Time:
5 minutes
Cook Time:
5 minutes
Serve: 4

Ingredients:

- 7 carrots, spiralized
- 2 tablespoons lime juice
- 1 tablespoon olive oil
- 1 teaspoon ground black pepper

Directions:

1. Preheat the olive oil in the skillet well.

2. Add carrot and ground black pepper.

3. Roast the carrot for 2-3 minutes.

4. Add lime juice, stir the carrot, and cook it for 2 minutes more.

Nutrition: 77 calories, 1g protein, 11.4g carbohydrates, 3.5g fat, 2.8g fiber, 0mg cholesterol, 75mg sodium, 354mg potassium.

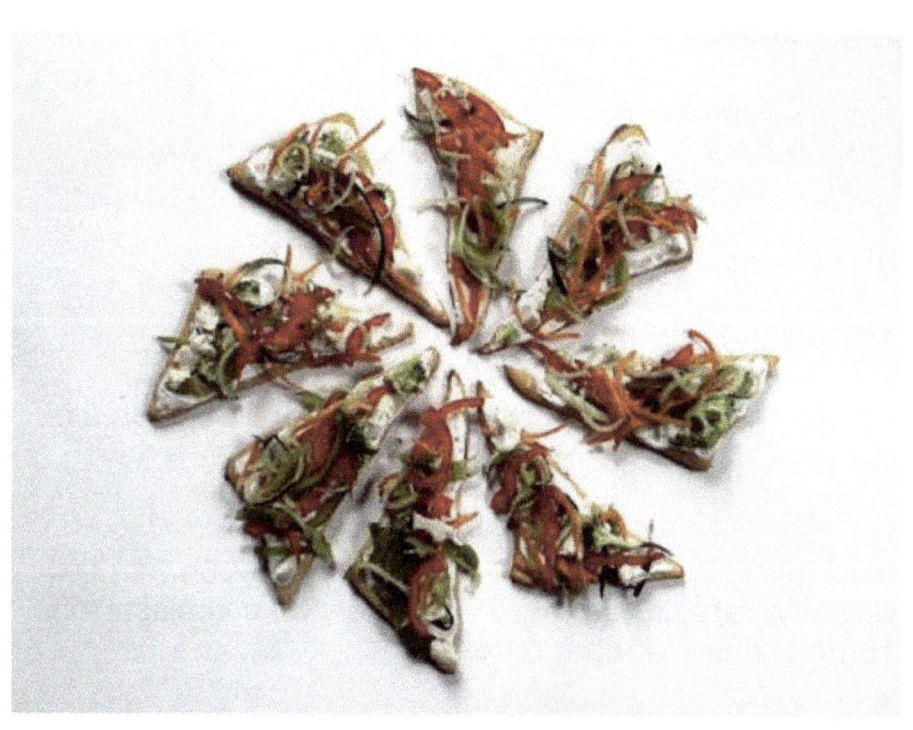

Classic Barley

Prep Time:
5 minutes
Cook Time:
30 minutes
Serve: 4

Ingredients:

- 2 cups barley
- 4 cups of water
- 1 tablespoon olive oil

Directions:

1. Mix water with barley and olive oil.

2. Cook the barley with the closed lid for 30 minutes on low heat.

Nutrition: 356 calories, 11.5g protein, 67.6g carbohydrates, 5.6g fat, 15.9g fiber, 0mg cholesterol, 18mg sodium, 418mg potassium.

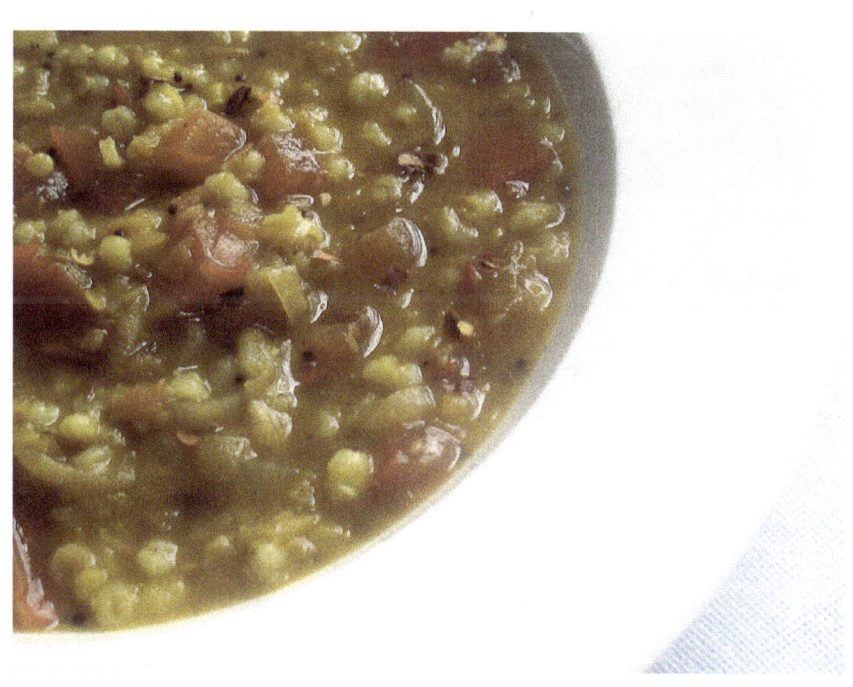

Baked Mango

Prep Time:
5 minutes
Cook Time:
20 minutes
Serve: 4

Ingredients:

- 2 mangos, peeled and chopped
- 1 tablespoon Italian seasonings
- 1 tablespoon olive oil

Directions:

1. Mix mango with Italian seasonings and olive oil.

2. Put the mango in the tray and bake it for 20 minutes at 355F.

Nutrition: 131 calories, 1.4g protein, 25.2g carbohydrates, 4.1g fat, 2.7g fiber, 0mg cholesterol, 2mg sodium, 282mg potassium.

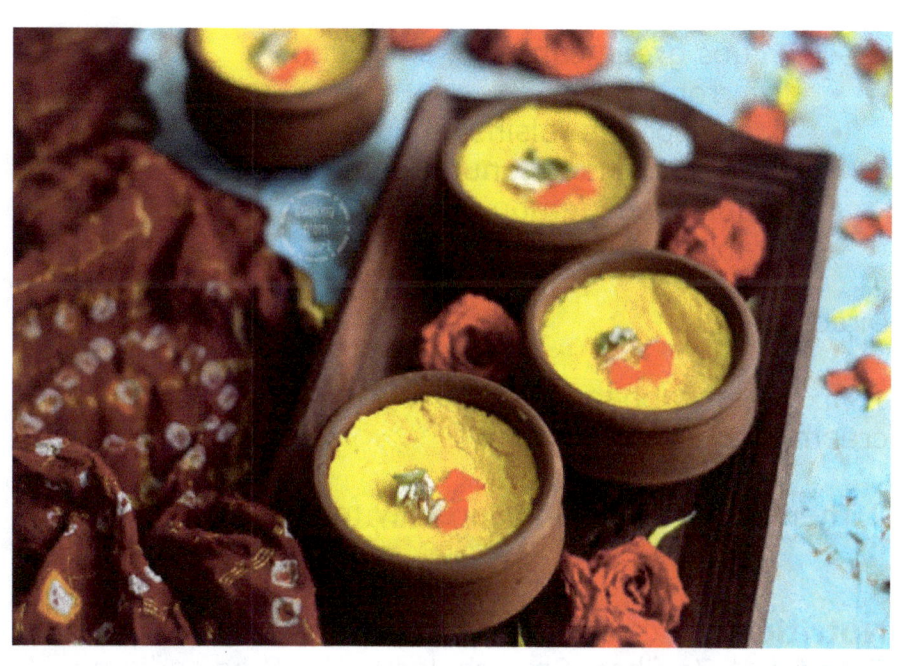

Easy Cabbage Slaw

Prep Time:
10 minutes
Cook Time:
0 minutes
Serve: 4

Ingredients:

- 2 cups green cabbage, shredded
- 1 carrot, grate
- 3 tablespoons raisins, chopped
- 2 tablespoons coconut cream
- 1 tablespoon lemon juice
- 1 tablespoon olive oil

Directions:

1. Mix green cabbage with carrot, raisins, coconut cream, and lemon juice.

2. Then add olive oil and carefully mix the slaw.

Nutrition: 83 calories, 1g protein, 9.4g carbohydrates, 5.4g fat, 1.7g fiber, 0mg cholesterol, 19mg sodium, 184mg potassium.

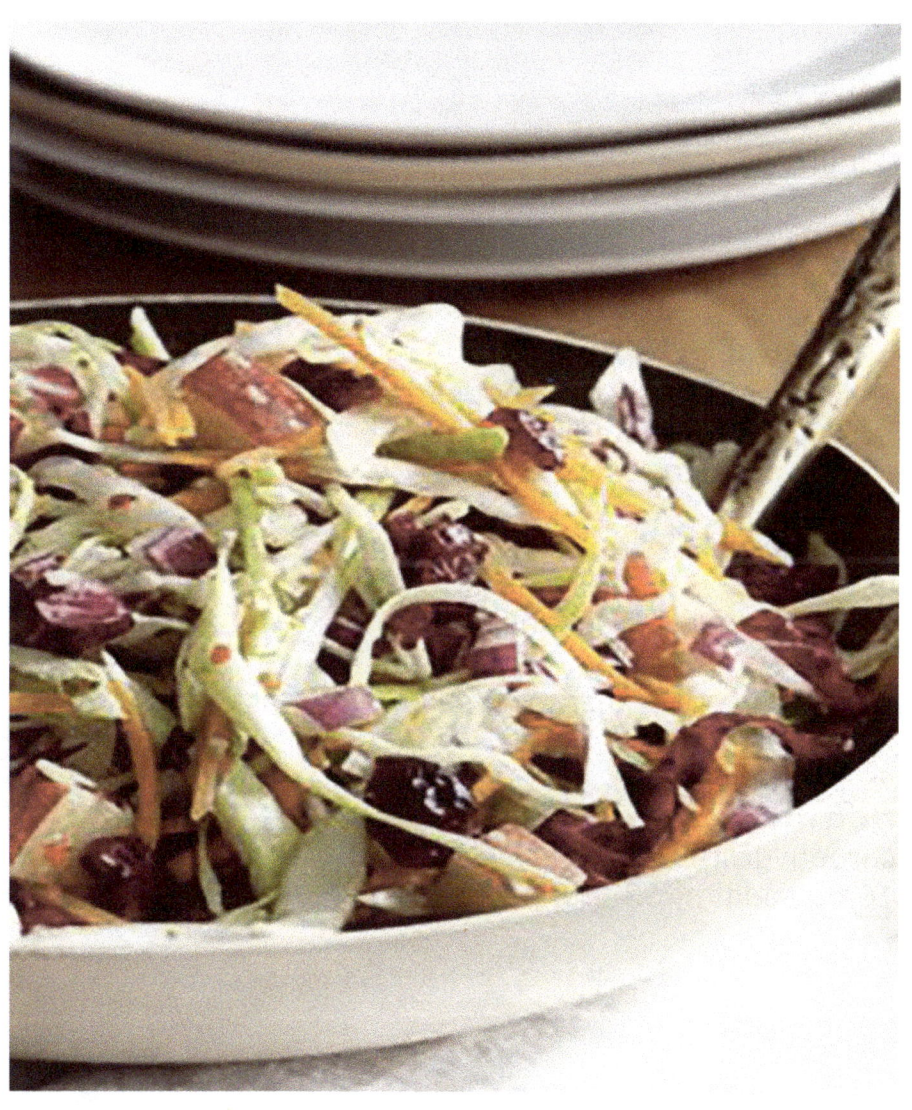

Apple Salad

Prep Time:
5 minutes
Cook Time:
0 minutes
Serve: 4

Ingredients:

- 5 apples, chopped
- ½ cup fresh dill, chopped
- 1 tablespoon olive oil
- 1 tomato, chopped

Directions:

1. Mix apples with dill and tomato.

2. Add olive oil and stir the salad one more time.

Nutrition: 193 calories, 2.1g protein, 42.5g carbohydrates, 4.3g fat, 7.8g fiber, 0mg cholesterol, 16mg sodium, 533mg potassium.

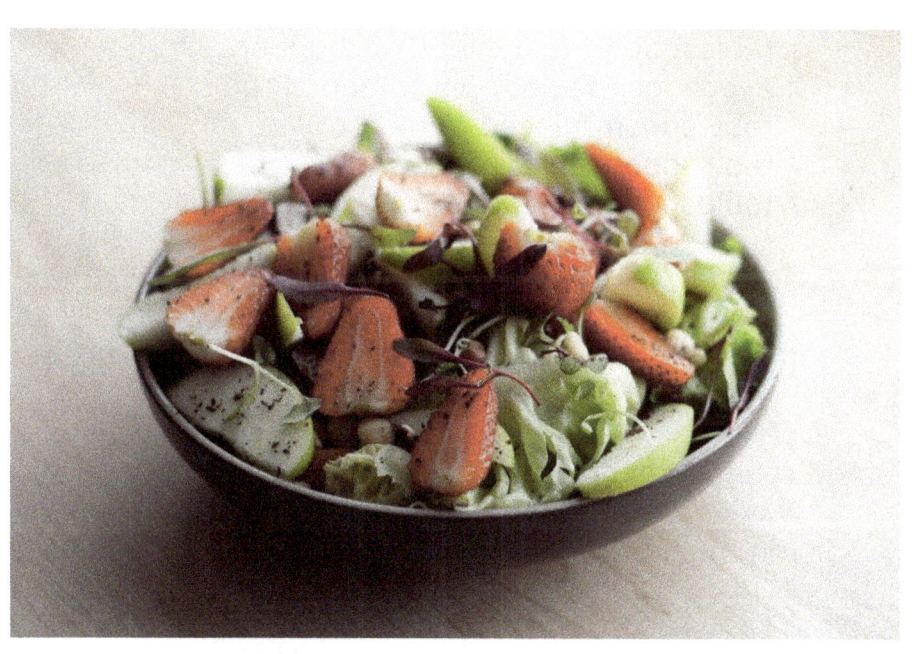

Avocado Mash

Prep Time:
10 minutes
Cook Time:
0 minutes
Serve: 4

Ingredients:

- 1 tablespoon fresh cilantro, chopped
- 2 avocados, peeled, pitted and sliced
- 1 tablespoon minced garlic
- 2 tablespoons lemon juice
- 1 tablespoon olive oil

Directions:

1. Blend the avocado until smooth and transfer it in the bowl.

2. Add cilantro, minced garlic, lemon juice, and olive oil.

3. Stir the meal well.

Nutrition: 240 calories, 2.1g protein, 9.5g carbohydrates, 23.2g fat, 6.8g fiber, 0mg cholesterol, 8mg sodium, 507mg potassium.

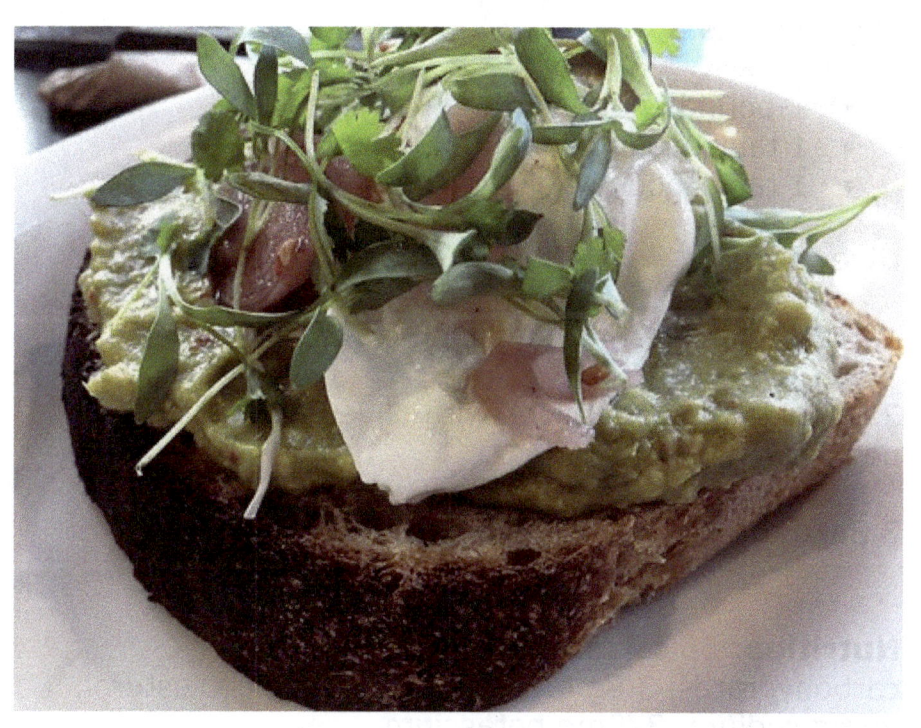

Bake Endives

Prep Time:
10 minutes
Cook Time:
20 minutes
Serve: 4

Ingredients:

- 1-pound endives, roughly chopped
- 1 tablespoon olive oil
- 1 tablespoon garlic powder

Directions:

1. Put the endives in the baking tray.

2. Sprinkle the vegetables with olive oil and garlic powder.

3. Bake the endives at 365F for 20 minutes.

Nutrition: 56 calories, 1.8g protein, 5.3g carbohydrates, 3.8g fat, 3.7g fiber, 0mg cholesterol, 26mg sodium, 379mg potassium.

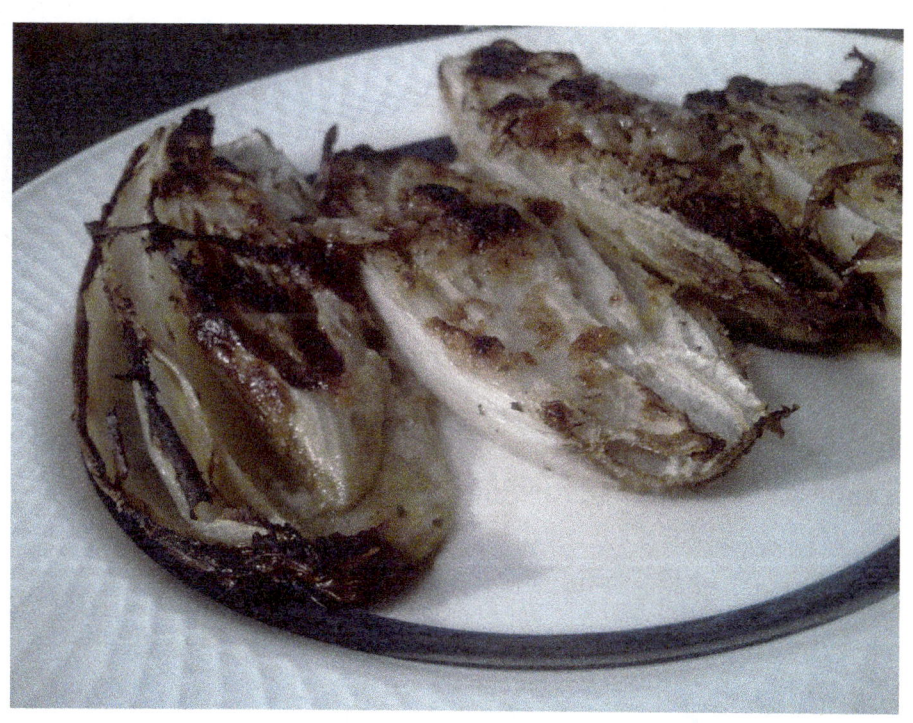

Arugula Bowl

Prep Time:
5 minutes
Cook Time:
0 minutes
Serve: 4

Ingredients:

- 2 cups baby arugula
- Juice of 1 lime
- 1 cup tomatoes, chopped
- 3 oz Romano cheese, crumbled
- 1 tablespoon olive oil

Directions:

1. Put all ingredients in the bowl.

2. Shake the meal before serving.

Nutrition: 128 calories, 7.7g protein, 4.6g carbohydrates, 9.4g fat, 1.2g fiber, 22mg cholesterol, 260mg sodium, 181mg potassium.

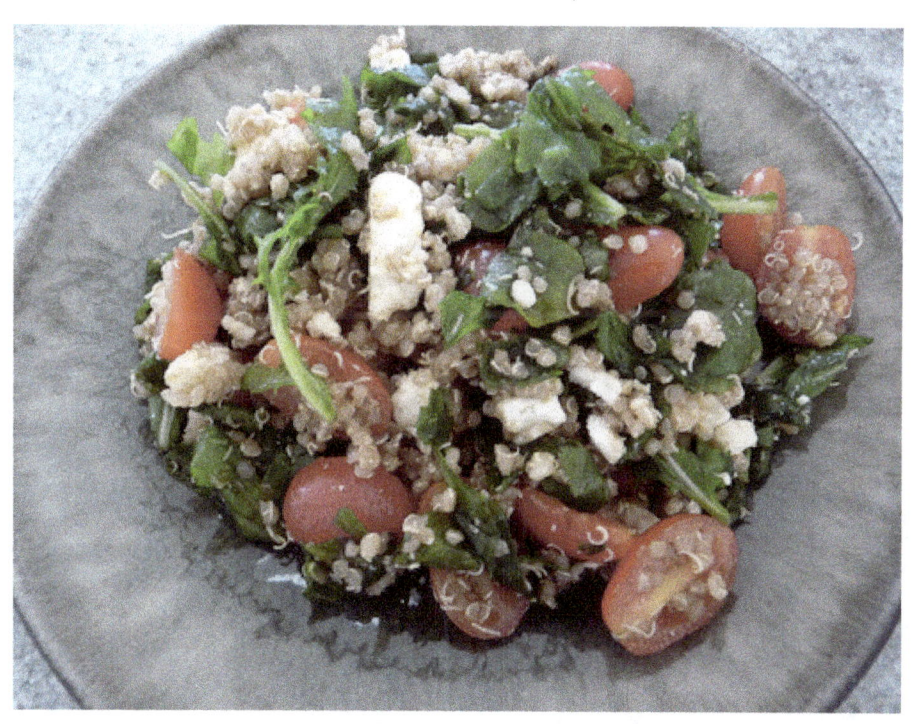

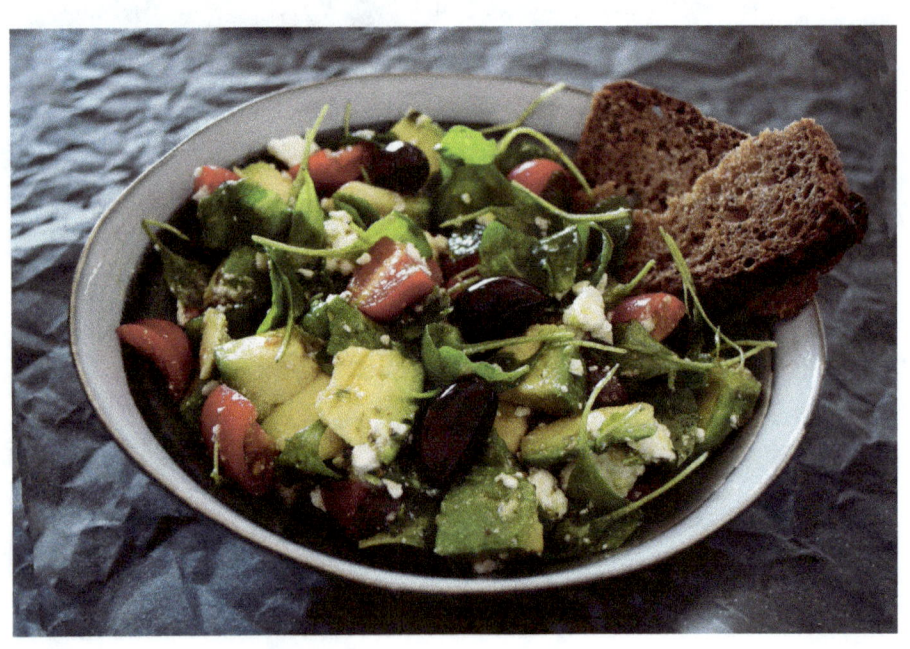

www.ingramcontent.com/pod-product-compliance
Lightning Source LLC
Chambersburg PA
CBHW070724030426
42336CB00013B/1914